Radiology of the Respiratory System

Christopher Flower, MB, B.CHIR, FRCP(C), FRCR

Consultant Radiologist
Addenbrooke's Hospital
Cambridge

Published,
in association with
UPDATE PUBLICATIONS LTD., by

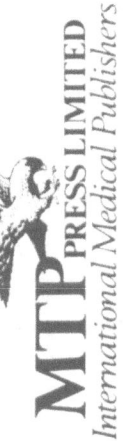

MTP PRESS LIMITED
International Medical Publishers

Published,
in association with
Update Publications Ltd., by

MTP Press Limited
Falcon House
Lancaster, England

Softcover reprint of the hardcover 1st edition 1981

First published 1981

ISBN-13: 978-94-009-8092-1   e-ISBN-13: 978-94-009-8090-7

DOI: 10.1007/978-94-009-8090-7

Contents

1. The Chest: Normal Techniques and Pitfalls in Diagnosis

The first step in the interpretation of a chest radiograph is the recognition of an abnormality. Lesions then must be localized in anatomical terms (for example, lung, pleura or mediastinum) and finally, if possible, a pathological diagnosis applied. Recognition of an abnormality presupposes the opportunity to view films of adequate radiographic technique and a thorough knowledge of the radiographic appearances of the normal chest.

Standard Radiographic Projections

The standard radiographic projections obtained are in the posteroanterior (PA) and lateral positions. Even slight rotation of the patient on the PA film may cause the heart and aorta to assume a peculiar configuration. One lung may appear relatively translucent and the hila

asymmetrical. The relative prominence of a hilum can often be ascribed to this cause or to a dorsal scoliosis which will produce a similar appearance. The simplest way to check the patient's position is to measure the distance between the medial ends of the clavicles and the adjacent dorsal spinous process. Thoracic deformities, such as pectus excavatum, may distort the mediastinal structures (Figure 1.1).

Posteroanterior View

On the PA view a large area of lung is obscured by the heart, great vessels and diaphragm. An adequately penetrated film is therefore essential to 'see through' the heart. Paravertebral masses and lesions in the posterior basal segment of the left lower lobe are then less likely to be missed. As a generalization it is better to have a dark film that can be viewed satisfactorily with a bright light, than too light a film which cannot provide the same information (Figures 1.2 and 1.3). Standard films are taken in full inspiration, and the diaphragm is normally seen opposite the posterior aspect of the 10th or 11th rib. Films taken with poor inspiration may be very misleading (Figure 1.4). Crowding of vessels in the lower lobes may simulate consolidation, particularly in children in whom the trachea may also assume a buckled appearance. Both costophrenic angles must be incorporated in the film if small pleural effusions are not to be missed.

1

2

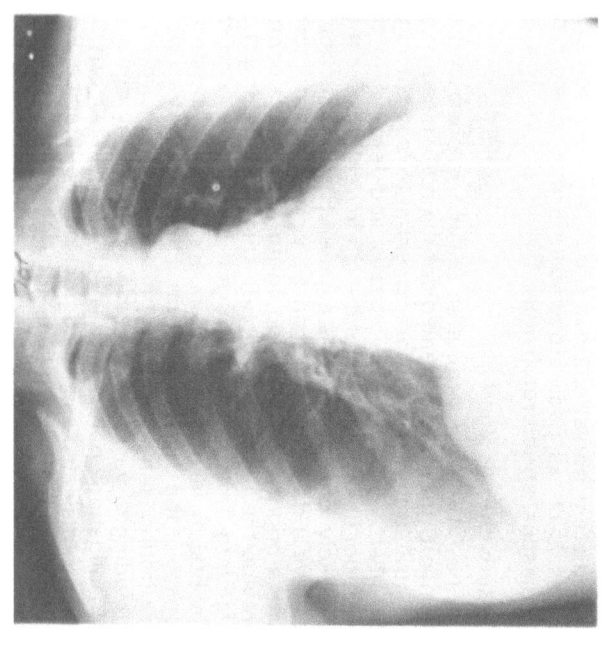

Figure 1.1. Advanced pectus excavatum causing mediastinal displacement and simulating cardiomegaly.

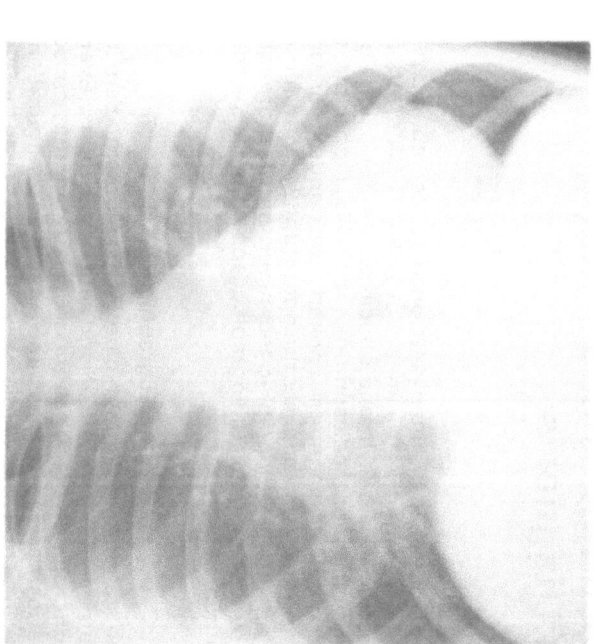

Figure 1.2. Underdeveloped film on which no abnormality can be detected.

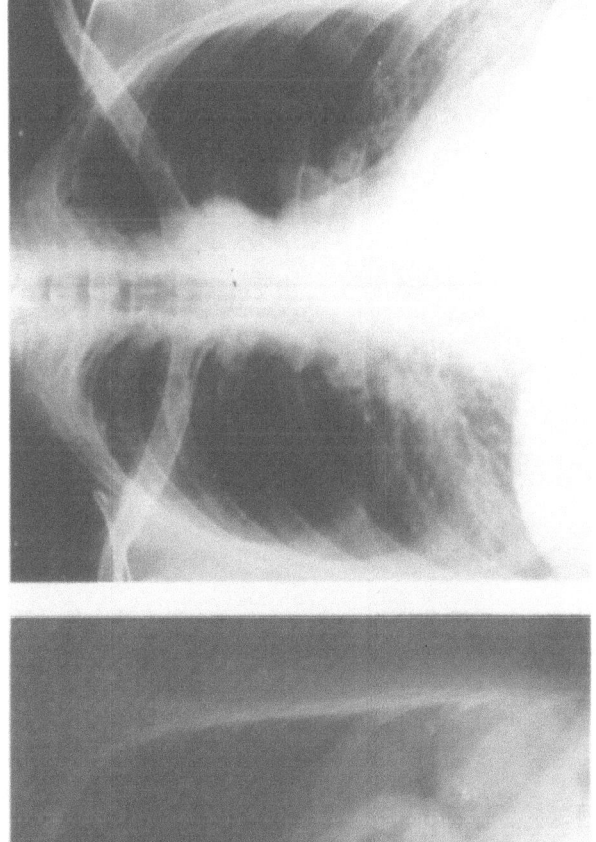

Figure 1.3. Same patient as in Figure 1.2. A slightly over-exposed film reveals a large hiatus hernia behind the heart.

Figure 1.4. Increased shadowing both lower zones due to crowding of the pulmonary vessels in a patient who has taken a poor inspiration.

3

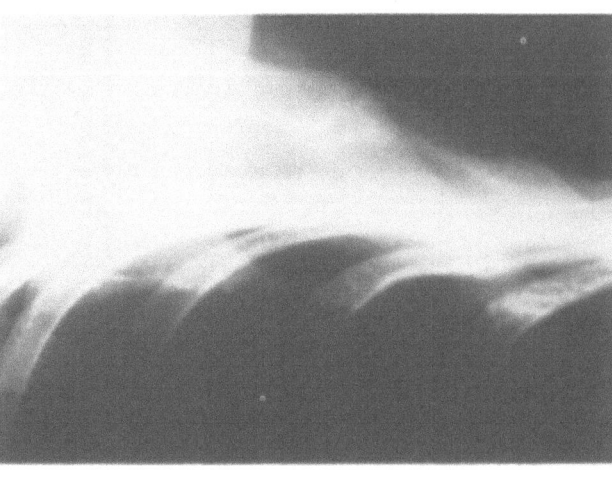

Figure 1.5. *A pseudofracture of the scapula, diagnostic of osteomalacia. The film was requested because the patient complained of tiredness and weight loss. The correct diagnosis was not initially suspected.*

Finally, no chest examination is complete unless the bones and soft tissues are analysed. Metastases are occasionally seen in the ribs and humeral necks; erosion of the outer aspects of the clavicles may provide evidence of hyperparathyroidism and pseudo-fractures of the rib indicate osteomalacia (Figure 1.5). The gastric air bubble is sometimes absent in achalasia of the cardia, while a proliferative carcinoma of the gastric fundus may be well outlined by air on the erect film. Free air or a fluid level beneath the diaphragm may provide evidence of a subphrenic abscess. A well penetrated, coned, erect film of the diaphragm may be required to visualize a small subphrenic abscess, as the routine erect chest radiograph is not satisfactory for this purpose.

It is axiomatic that a routine system of observation, which incorporates all aspects of the film, is scrupulously followed. A second look at the areas partially obscured by the clavicles and heart is worthwhile.

Some localization of an abnormality is occasionally permitted by scrutiny of the PA film alone. Intrapulmonary lesions at the level of the clavicle lie at the apex of the lung; while local rib erosion or destruction implies that the lesion is adjacent to it. A further very helpful aid to localization is the 'silhouette sign', described by Felson. It is based on the observation that an intrathoracic opacity abutting against the border of the heart, aorta, pulmonary artery or diaphragm should obliterate that border and *ipso facto* the converse holds (Figures 1.6 to 1.8). It is especially valuable in detecting middle and lower lobe disease (the latter may be more obvious on the PA than the lateral view) and sometimes in differentiating hilar masses from superimposed pulmonary or pleural lesions.

Localization of a lesion is not a purely academic exercise. It is obviously important if any form of surgical intervention or biopsy procedure is likely, and it may also provide an important clue to the pathological nature of the lesion. Thus, an anterior cavity is unlikely to be tuberculous, an opacity adjacent to the aorta may be vascular in nature, a recurrent pneumonia in the apical segment of the lower lobe may be caused by aspiration. Much of the lung is hidden on the PA film, and it can reasonably be argued that a lateral view is mandatory. This ideal is not always possible which makes the preceding comments concerning observations made from the PA film alone all the more important.

Lateral View

It is customary to obtain that lateral view which places the side containing the lesion nearest to the film. When viewing the film a routine system of observation should be applied, as with the PA film. The retrosternal and retrocardiac spaces are usually of roughly equal

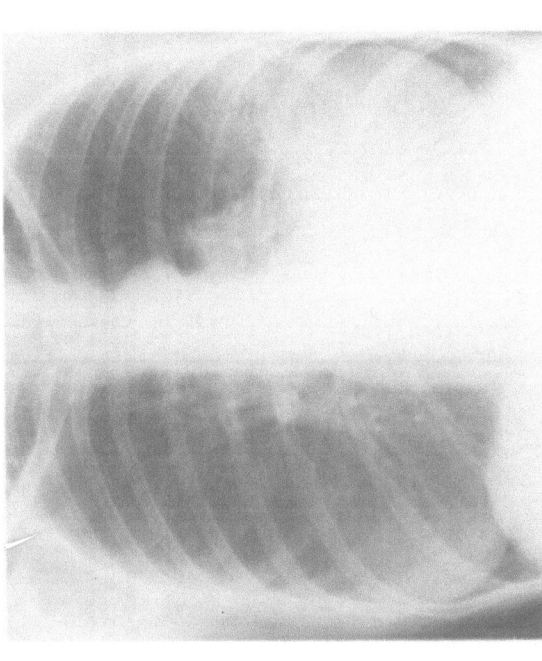

Figure 1.6. *Lingular pneumonia, producing consolidation which obliterates the left heart border.*

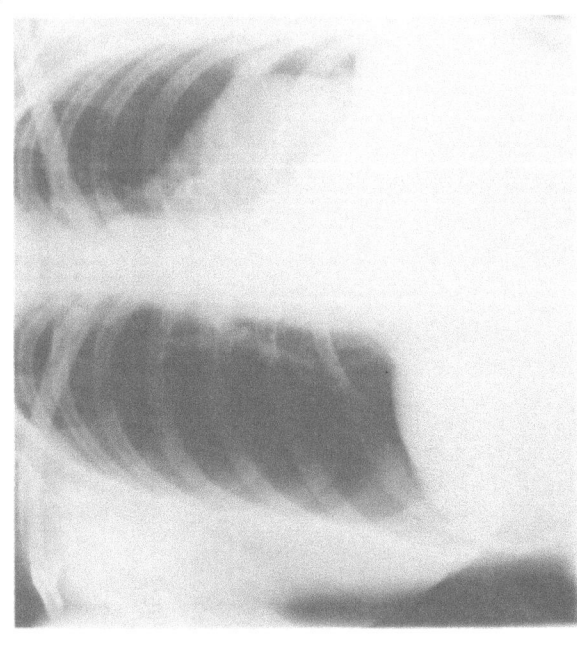

Figure 1.7. The lateral film of the same patient as in Figure 1.6 confirms that the consolidation lies in the anterior aspect of the chest, in the lingula.

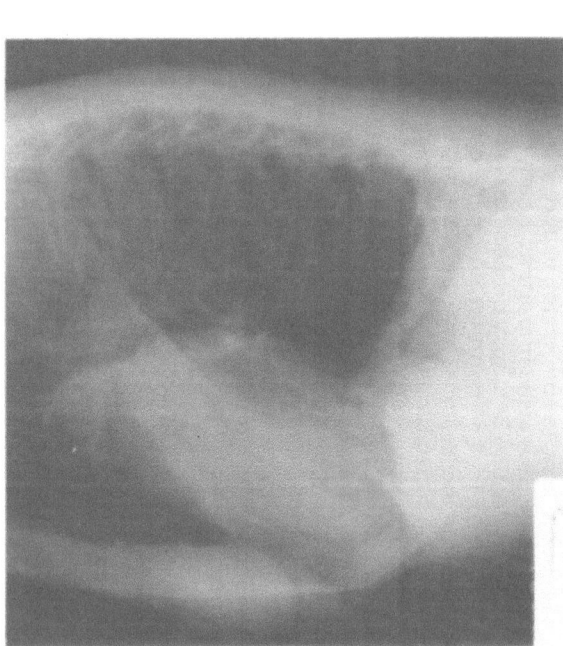

Figure 1.8. There is an opacity adjacent to, but not obliterating, the left heart border on this PA film. The lesion should therefore lie posteriorly. The lateral film confirmed this.

size and translucency. In keeping with this, the dorsal vertebral bodies increase in translucency as one reaches the diaphragm. If this is not seen, lower lobe disease is likely.

The hemidiaphragms can usually be differentiated by their relative heights and configurations and by the air-filled gastric fundus adjacent to the left leaf. Both leaves should be entirely clear, except where the left leaf meets the heart. Any loss of definition implies the presence of adjacent disease, such as pneumonia or tumour. Both the costovertebral and costophrenic angles should be acute. Blunting of either angle may be the first evidence of a pleural effusion. Pericardial and valve calcification (both aortic and mitral) are usually best seen on a lateral view, and indeed may be completely missed on the PA projection. The lateral film also helps to elucidate the intrathoracic position of such opacities as mediastinal masses, and lobar and segmental collapse, and it may be the only film of the two views on which a lesion is seen (Figures 1.9 and 1.10). It is occasionally true that the lateral film will be quite unhelpful. For example, it may appear surprisingly normal in complete lower lobe collapse. As with the PA film, it is worth having a second look at certain areas, e.g. the retrosternal space and the infrahilar region.

Having observed and then localized an abnormality, an attempt must be made to apply a pathological

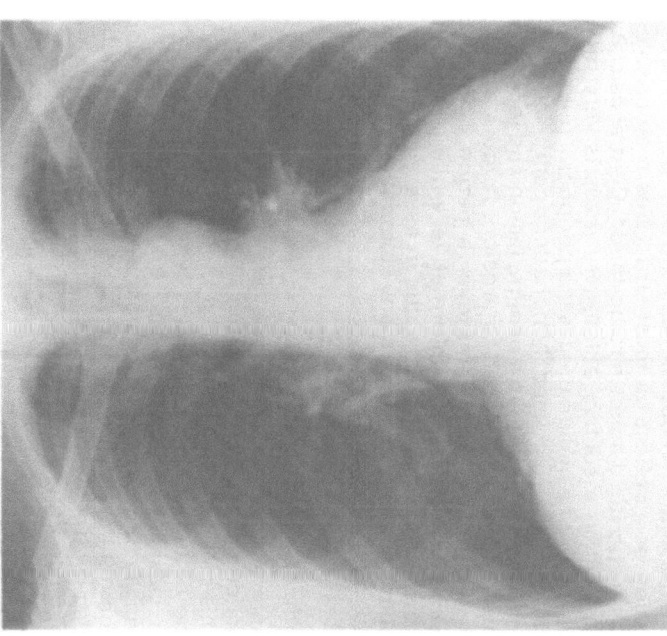

Figure 1.9. *No abnormality is seen on this PA radiograph.*

diagnosis. This is frequently not possible from a single examination, but occasionally the configuration of the lesion or its effect on local structures may enable a fairly specific diagnosis to be made. Central calcification within a solitary pulmonary mass is very much in favour of a benign process; a peripheral pulmonary cavity with associated lymphadenopathy favours a malignant, rather than a benign, lesion and local bony destruction, as opposed to erosion, favours a malignant process. Serial films over a period of days or weeks will often prove informative, while recourse to previous films is of great value in assessing a solitary pulmonary mass and many examples of diffuse pulmonary shadowing.

Other Radiographic Views

Anteroposterior (AP) views are often obtained in preference to the PA view in ill patients or children. This may also be a valuable projection in determining the nature of small opacities which overlie the ribs or clavicles on the standard PA film, as these are usually thrown clear of the bones on the AP projection. The main deficiency of the AP view is the inevitable distortion of the mediastinal structures which are some distance from the film. Thus, there may be apparent cardiomegaly or a widened superior mediastinum when no such abnormality exists.

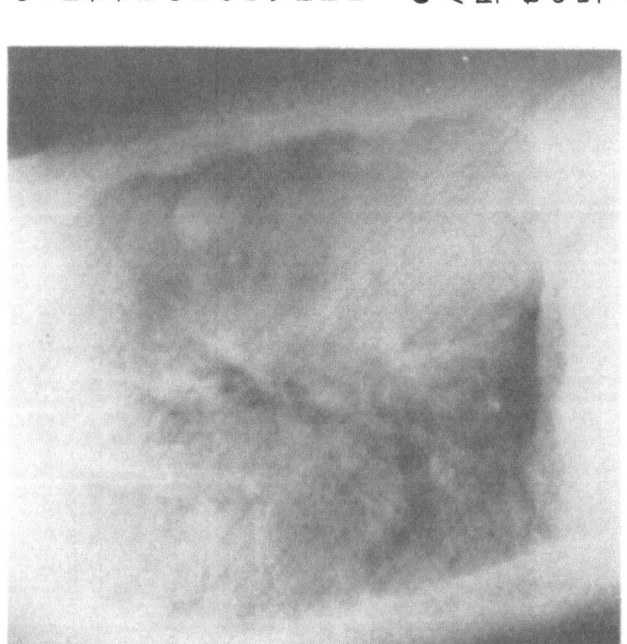

Figure 1.10. The lateral film reveals a 2 cm opacity in the anterior segment of the left upper lobe. It overlies the left hilum on the PA film but occupies the retrosternal space on the lateral film.

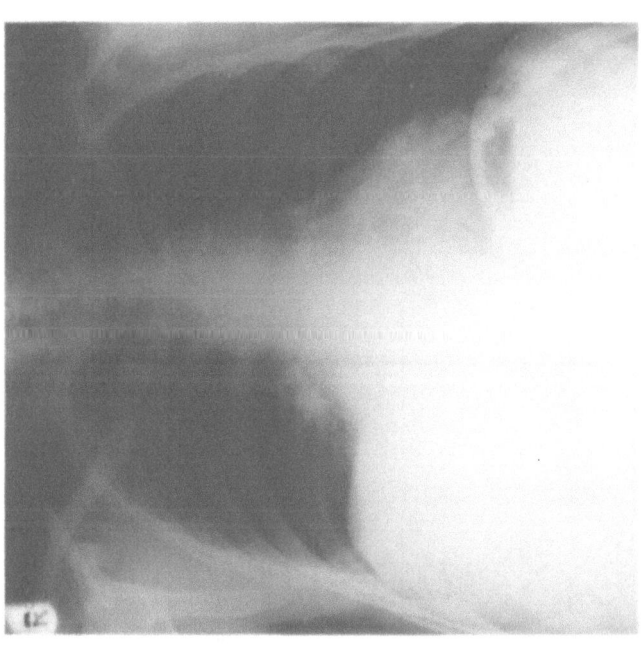

Supine views produce greater distortion of the mediastinum. It is often difficult for the patient to take a full inspiration. This view is very much a second best examination, although occasionally it can be most useful in establishing the vascular nature of a pulmonary or mediastinal mass. Thus, an arteriovenous malformation may be differentiated from a solid tumour and the azygos vein from an enlarged lymph node at the tracheobronchial angle. Subpulmonary collections of fluid, mimicking a high hemidiaphragm, will also be demonstrated in this position (Figures 1.11 and 1.12).

Smaller collections of pleural fluid will usually require decubitus views, without which it is often difficult to differentiate fluid from pleural thickening. As little as 200 ml fluid can be demonstrated if care is taken to obtain good films.

The importance of a good inspiratory film has already been mentioned. Films in expiration may be of immense value in demonstrating a small pneumothorax and 'air trapping'. The latter may occur distal to any main, lobar or segmental bronchial occlusion. Expiratory films should never be omitted if there is a history of foreign body aspiration in a child (Figures 1.13 and 1.14). It is sometimes rewarding in an adult presenting with a wheeze in whom the inspiratory film is normal (Figures 1.15 and 1.16).

Figure 1.11. *The erect film suggests that there is elevation of the right hemidiaphragm. However, note its slightly unusual configuration.*

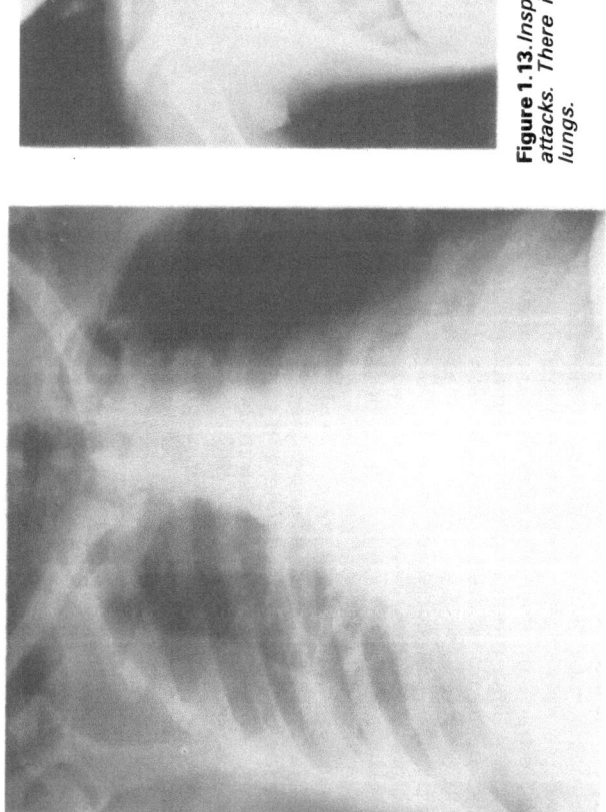

Figure 1.13. Inspiratory film of a child with a history of choking attacks. There is little difference in the appearance of the lungs.

Figure 1.12. A supine film. The pleural fluid which was subpulmonary in position, occupies the posterior aspect of the right hemithorax, which is rendered more opaque.

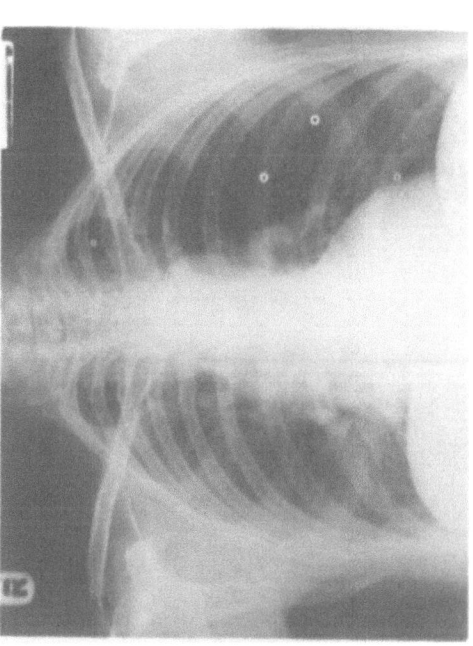

Figure 1.14. *An expiratory film reveals a hyperlucent left lung, related to air trapping due to a peanut lodged in the left main bronchus.*

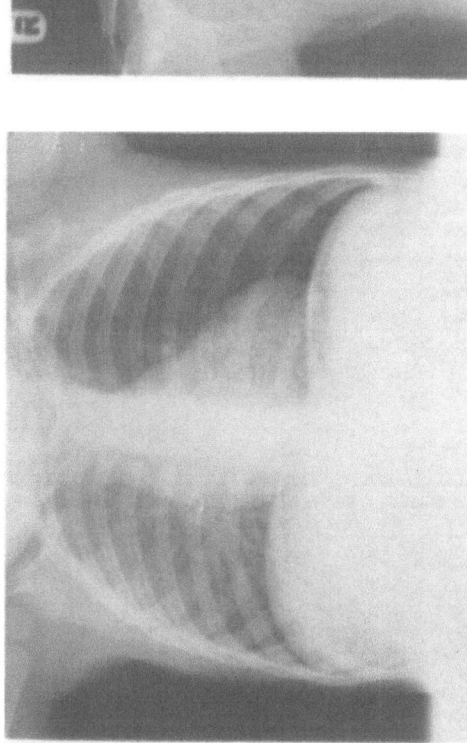

Figure 1.15. *An expiratory film of a patient who complained of wheezing reveals a slightly more transradiant and larger left lung than normal due to air trapping.*

A lordotic view is taken with a horizontal beam, but with the back arched. It is commonly used for better visualization of the apical regions of the upper lobes, giving a more bone-free, albeit distorted, view (Figures 1.17 and 1.18). It is also a graphic method of confirming right middle lobe collapse (see Figure 4.11).

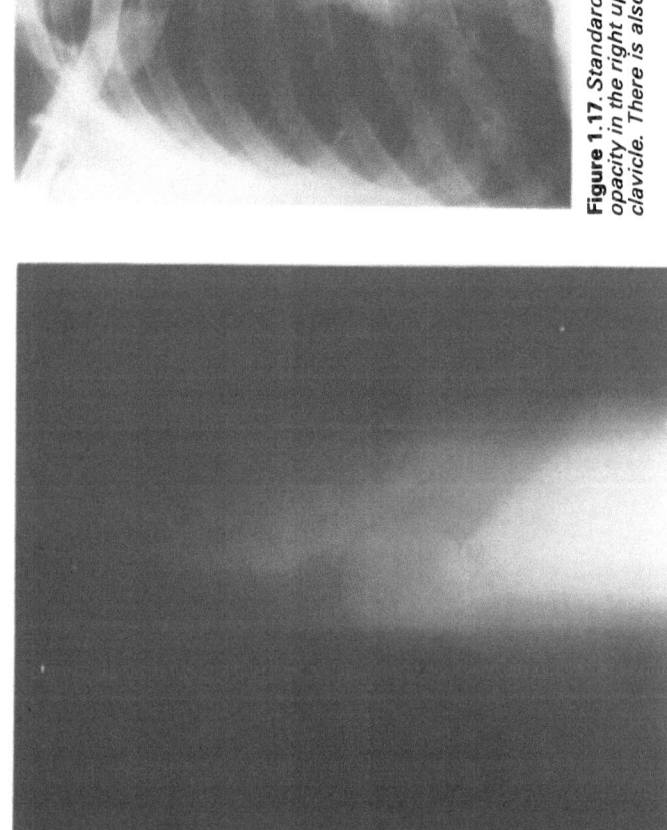

Figure 1.16. *A mediastinal tomogram reveals a polypoid tumour at the carina almost occluding the left main bronchus.*

Figure 1.17. *Standard PA radiograph. There is a questionable opacity in the right upper lobe overlapped by the first rib and clavicle. There is also left lower lobe pneumonia.*

and not pulsatile, while masses adjacent to the aorta or pulmonary arteries often exhibit marked transmitted pulsations. The large, 'quiet' heart of a pericardial effusion may be simulated by the large heart of advanced myocardial ischaemia and by a cardiomyopathy. Fluoroscopy is of value in the assessment of diaphragmatic function (see Chapter 10), although it should be remembered that a high, immobile diaphragm does not necessarily indicate phrenic nerve paralysis. Adjacent pulmonary or pleural disease may render the adjacent diaphragmatic leaf relatively immobile, as may subdiaphragmatic suppurations. Mitral and aortic valve calcification may be recognized and distinguished by careful fluoroscopy in the oblique or lateral projection.

Fluoroscopy is invaluable in two situations: in the differentiation of a normal thymic shadow from other lesions in the infant and young child, and in the correct localization of an intrathoracic lesion. In the latter case, it is an excellent method of differentiating intrapulmonary from pleural and chest wall tumours.

Tomography

Tomography is a valuable means of obtaining better definition of an intrathoracic opacity. It is most commonly used with pulmonary and mediastinal masses. The margins are well delineated, and any cavitation or calcification within the lesion, invisible

13

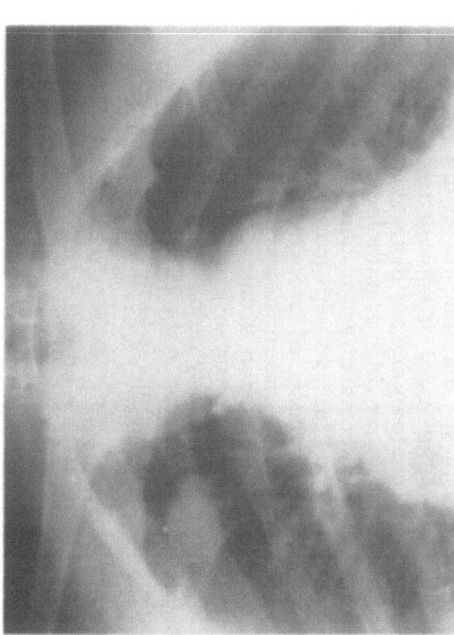

Figure 1.18. *An apical lordotic view confirms the presence of a 2 cm opacity (carcinoma).*

Other Radiological Techniques

Fluoroscopy

The classical use of fluoroscopy is in the differentiation of vascular from non-vascular lesions, which is often very difficult in practice. Aneurysms may be full of clot

on the routine films, will usually be seen. It is extremely useful in the evaluation of doubtful hilar enlargement and in the assessment of the mediastinum for enlarged nodes.

Bronchography

Bronchography is much less commonly employed than previously. It is usually performed by the transnasal or transcricoid route, but is increasingly undertaken via the flexible bronchoscope. Local anaesthesia is used except in children, for whom a general anaesthetic is necessary. It demonstrates accurately the bronchial anatomy and any distortion of it, but does not necessarily provide a pathological diagnosis. Bronchoscopy allows direct visualization of all the major segmental bronchi with the added benefits of biopsy. The diagnosis of bronchiectasis is usually obvious on clinical grounds, and bronchography is only occasionally needed as corroborative evidence. It may also be required for assessment of the extent of the disease, particularly before surgery. Bronchography is now rarely used in the evaluation of peripheral pulmonary lesions; this is better achieved by biopsy.

Biopsy

Percutaneous needle biopsy is a proven method of establishing the diagnosis of a well defined peripheral pulmonary lesion. It requires good cytological

facilities, when the accuracy for the diagnosis of malignant lesions is between 80 and 90 per cent. It is a less satisfactory method for dealing with more ill defined peripheral shadows, which are better approached via a flexible bronchoscope. Image intensification is mandatory for percutaneous needle biopsy and is a very helpful aid when biopsying peripheral masses via the flexible bronchoscope.

Pulmonary Angiography

Pulmonary angiography is the ideal method for the investigation and diagnosis of intrapulmonary vascular abnormalities, such as arteriovenous malformations and pulmonary artery aneurysms. It is also used in the diagnosis of pulmonary embolism (see Chapter 6) and certain rarities of the pulmonary vasculature, such as primary pulmonary hypertension and veno-occlusive disease.

Thoracic Aortography

Thoracic aortography is most commonly used for, and is often invaluable in, the diagnosis of mediastinal aortic aneurysms. It is also required to establish the diagnosis of aortic dissection and rupture.

Bronchial Arteriography

Bronchial arteriography is sometimes used in the assessment of rare congenital heart lesions (e.g.

pulmonary atresia) and in the management of re-current haemoptysis when this is due to systemic–pulmonary shunts. These are occasionally congenital, but are more commonly acquired, usually from chronic inflammatory conditions, such as tuberculosis and bronchiectasis.

Computerized Axial Tomography

Computerized axial tomography now plays an increasingly important role in the management of

intrathoracic malignancy. It is particularly useful in assessing mediastinal masses and in demonstrating small pulmonary metastases and pleural masses.

Ultrasound

The major use of ultrasound in the chest is echocardiography. It is also an invaluable aid to the diagnosis of subphrenic abscesses and the differentiation of pleural effusions from thickened pleura or pleural tumours. It readily allows localization of pleural fluid prior to aspiration.

2. The Abnormal Hilum

Abnormalities of one or both hila pose a frequent diagnostic problem. Before discussing the causes of such abnormalities, it is pertinent to review the anatomy of the normal hilar shadow. This is produced by the main pulmonary arteries and their bifurcations and the upper lobe veins. The bronchi, which are air-containing and the lower lobe pulmonary veins, which pass inferiorly, form no component of the normal hilar shadow. Lymph nodes only contribute to the shadow when enlarged (Figure 2.1).

It is important to be thoroughly conversant with the normal size, shape and position of each hilum. Although, in any particular individual, the hila are usually of roughly equal dimensions, hilar size varies, often quite considerably, from one individual to another. For this reason standardized methods of measurement are of no practical use. Each hilum normally has a concave lateral aspect (Figure 2.1), and both are normally of equal radio-opacity. Any loss of the lateral concavity, a difference in their relative opacities, or loss of sharpness may be early evidence

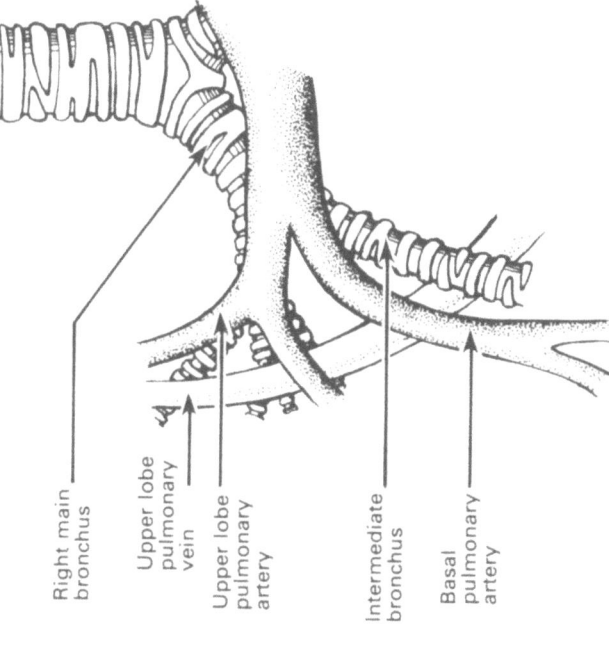

Right main bronchus

Upper lobe pulmonary vein

Upper lobe pulmonary artery

Intermediate bronchus

Basal pulmonary artery

Figure 2.1. *Diagrammatic representation of the normal right hilum.*

of disease. The left hilum normally lies higher than the right. This is related to the fact that the left main bronchus (hyparterial) passes below the left main pulmonary artery, while the right main bronchus (eparterial) passes above the right main pulmonary artery.

The PA Film

All the preceding comments concern the PA film, which is of most value in assessing the hilar shadow. These important features can only be appreciated in properly performed and adequately penetrated radiographs. A questionably abnormal hilum is all too frequently related to inadequate radiographic technique. Patient rotation and dorsal scoliosis are common dissemblers (Figure 2.2). A hilar mass should never be diagnosed without viewing a lateral film – it is invaluable in distinguishing true from apparent hilar enlargement, because of a superimposed lesion in the lung, pleura or chest wall (Figures 2.3 and 2.4). Coned, well penetrated films and careful fluoroscopy can yield further information, but tomography, in AP, oblique and lateral projections, is the most useful additional examination. In most instances, this allows one to differentiate between normal and abnormal shadows and to distinguish between solid and vascular lesions. Hilar calcification is well seen and bronchial patency may be assessed (Figures 2.5 and 2.6).

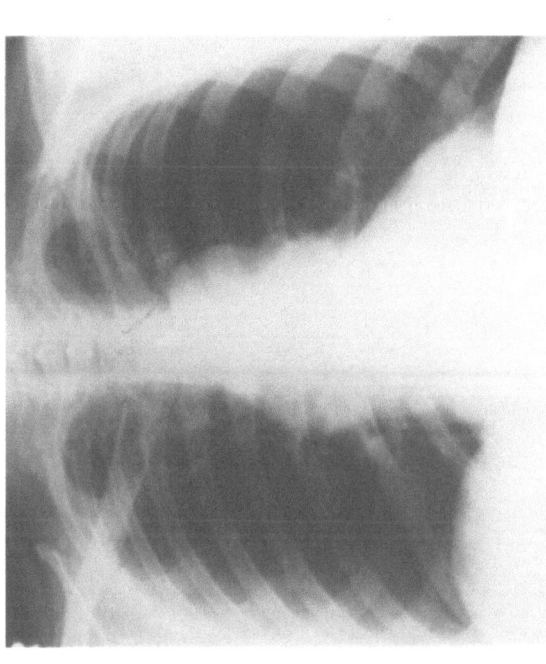

Figure 2.2. *The combination of patient rotation and an un-folded aorta simulates right hilar enlargement.*

It is most convenient to consider the causes of hilar abnormalities according to enlargement or diminution in size (Tables 2.1 and 2.2).

17

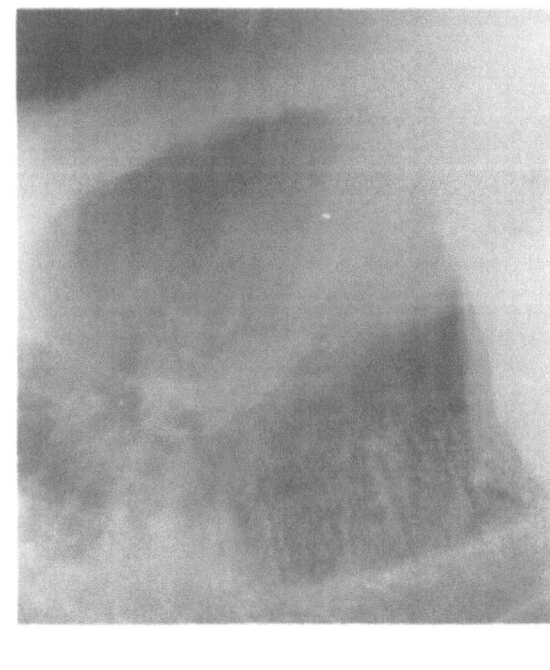

Figure 2.4. The lateral film reveals consolidation in the apical segment of the left lower lobe, directly behind the hilum, which is normal.

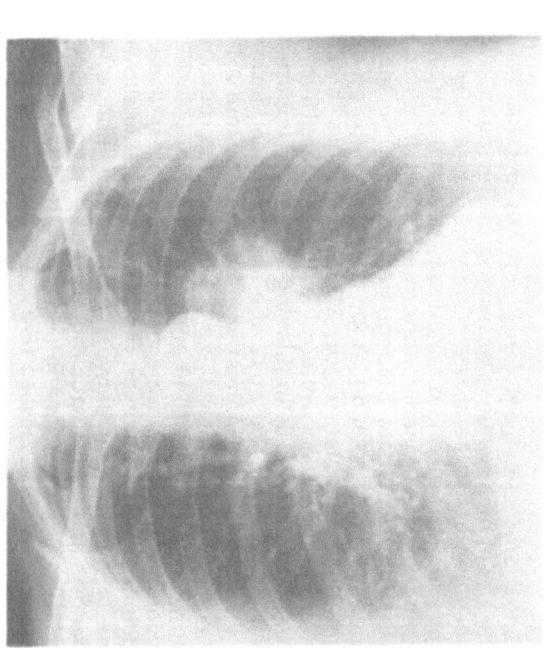

Figure 2.3. The PA film suggests enlargement of the left hilum.

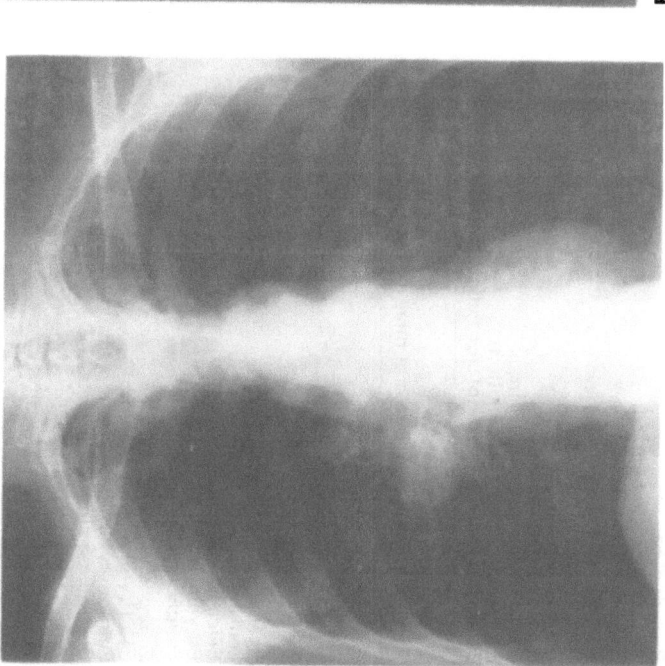

Figure 2.5. Bronchial carcinoma causing enlargement of the lower pole of the right hilum.

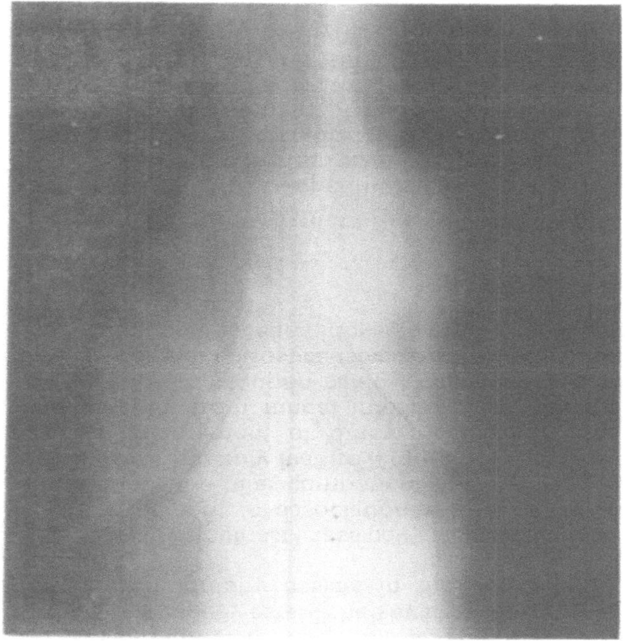

Figure 2.6. A tomogram of a patient with a carcinoma at the right hilum reveals narrowing of the right main bronchus (retouched).

19

Table 2.1. Causes of unilateral hilar enlargement.

Bronchial carcinoma
Metastatic malignancy
Lymphomas
Primary tuberculosis
Fungal infections
Sarcoidosis
Pulmonary embolism
Pulmonary artery aneurysm
Pulmonary valve stenosis (left)
Following Blalock operation for Fallot's tetralogy

Table 2.2. Causes of bilateral hilar enlargement.

Enlarged lymph nodes
Lymphomas
Sarcoidosis
Metastatic malignancy
Cystic fibrosis
Infectious mononucleosis
Leukaemia
Silicosis
Berylliosis
Fungal infections
Enlarged vessels
Left to right cardiac shunts
Pulmonary arterial hypertension
Obstructive airways disease
Left heart failure
Pulmonary embolism
Polycythaemia rubra vera

Unilateral Hilar Enlargement

A proximal bronchial carcinoma is by far the commonest cause of unilateral hilar enlargement (Figure 2.5). Diagnosis is usually established by bronchoscopy with biopsy. Tomography assists in the assessment of operability.

Primary tuberculosis classically causes unilateral hilar enlargement in association with a pulmonary infiltrate, but the hilar component may be the most prominent or the only feature (Figure 2.7). There may also be enlargement of other mediastinal nodes. Differentiation from fungal infections is impossible and depends more upon clinical circumstances and local environment. Most causes listed in Table 2.1 are rare. It is unusual for sarcoidosis to produce unilateral hilar lymphadenopathy.

Bilateral Hilar Enlargement due to Large Nodes

Hodgkin's lymphoma frequently causes bilateral nodal enlargement, which is often asymmetrical (Figure 2.8). This is in contrast to sarcoidosis, where there is usually symmetrical enlargement of the bronchopulmonary nodes (Figure 2.9).

Hodgkin's disease and sarcoidosis may have an associated paratracheal lymphadenopathy. This is more common in Hodgkin's disease, where it may

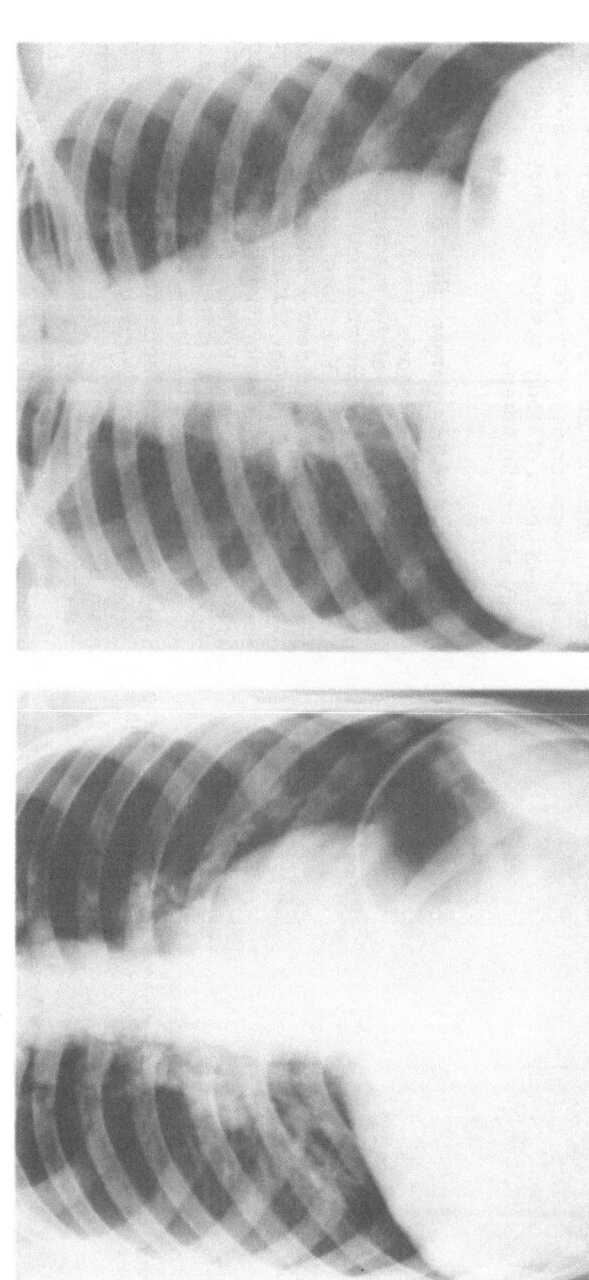

Figure 2.7. Primary tuberculosis causing enlargement of the right hilar lymph nodes.

Figure 2.8. Asymmetrical enlargement of bronchopulmonary and paratracheal nodes in a patient with Hodgkin's lymphoma.

21

occur without any associated hilar adenopathy (unlike sarcoidosis where the hilar component is more conspicuous). It is sometimes impossible to differentiate these two disorders by radiography alone.

Calcification of enlarged nodes may occur in silicosis (when it assumes an 'eggshell' appearance), and in cases of sarcoidosis, often with hypercalcaemia. The enlarged nodes of Hodgkin's disease may sometimes calcify after radiotherapy.

Bilateral Hilar Enlargement due to Large Vessels

Pulmonary valve stenosis usually only produces post-stenotic dilatation of the main pulmonary artery but this occasionally extends to the left pulmonary artery (Figure 2.10). The rare pulmonary artery aneurysm is only confidently diagnosed by angiographic means. Dilatation of the main pulmonary arteries is part of the generalized pulmonary plethora in left to right shunts. It is most pronounced in atrial septal defects (Figure 2.11). It is difficult to diagnose the presence or to assess the degree of pulmonary hypertension from the appearance of the vessels. In chronic bronchitis and emphysema dilatation of the main pulmonary artery and its major hilar branches is a common, albeit a very variable, accompaniment. The hilar shadows become more opaque, slightly larger and less well-defined in early left heart failure,

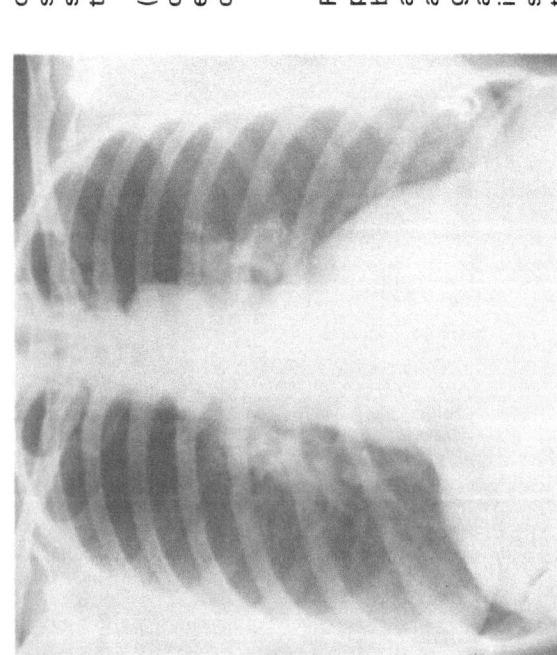

Figure 2.9. Symmetrical enlargement of the bronchopulmonary nodes at both hila in a patient with sarcoidosis.

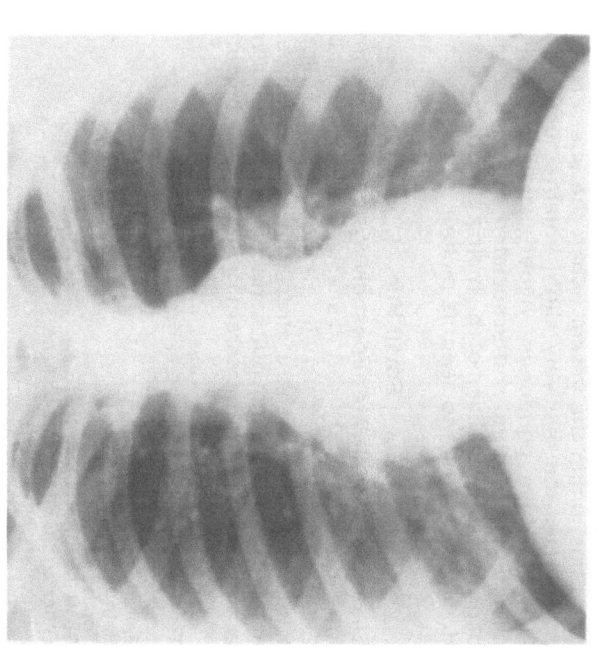

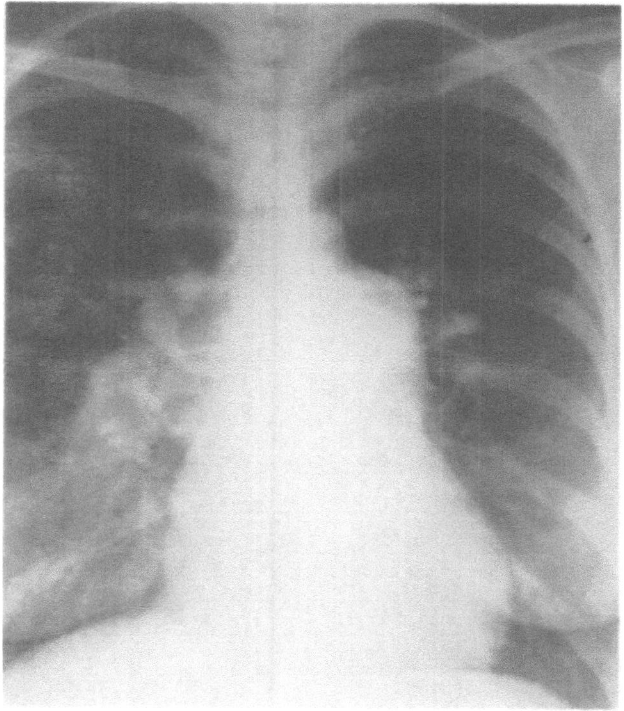

Figure 2.10. Enlargement of the main and left main pulmonary arteries in a patient with pulmonary valve stenosis.

Figure 2.11. Bilateral hilar enlargement due to increased size of the main pulmonary arteries in a patient with an atrial septal defect.

due to engorgement of the interstitial spaces with transudate; the dilated upper lobe veins are an added component of the enlarged hilum. Pulmonary embolism may lead to dilatation of one or both of the pulmonary arteries. This may be caused either by thrombus within the vessel (when the sharp cut-off accentuates the relatively slight enlargement) or by acute massive pulmonary hypertension, when the dilatation is bilateral and associated with pulmonary oligaemia and dilatation of the main pulmonary artery. However, it is rare to see this picture.

Small Hila

Bilateral small hila are almost always caused by some form of congenital heart disease (Table 2.3; Figure 2.12). The patient is usually cyanosed, and Fallot's tetralogy and pulmonary atresia are the commonest in this group. Although pulmonary thromboembolism is a cause of both unilateral (Table 2.4) and bilateral

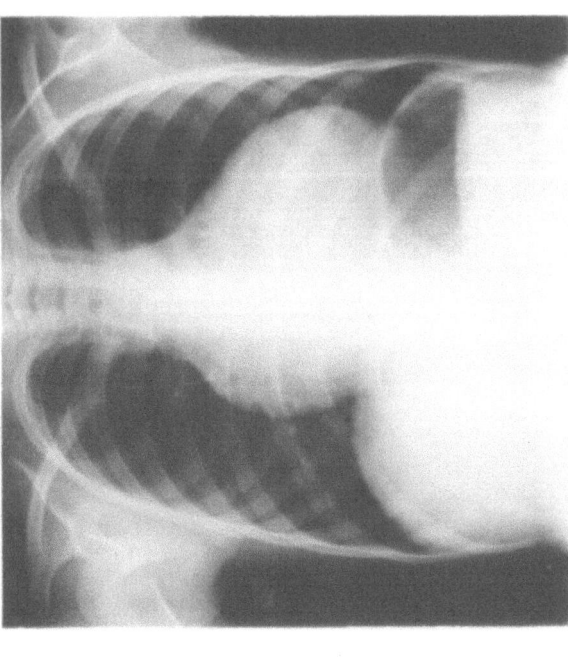

Figure 2.12. *Ebstein's anomaly. The small hilar shadows reflect the generalized pulmonary oligaemia.*

Table 2.3. Causes of bilateral decrease in hilar size.

Fallot's tetralogy
Pulmonary atresia
Tricuspid atresia
Ebstein's anomaly
Other congenital heart disease
Pulmonary embolism

Table 2.4. Causes of unilateral decrease in hilar size.

Lower lobe collapse
Pulmonary thromboembolism
Congenital hypoplasia of the pulmonary artery
Macleod's syndrome

decrease in hilar size, convincing plain film evidence of hilar abnormality is infrequent when one considers how common the condition is. The hilum usually appears small and displaced downwards in lower lobe collapse (Figure 4.6). Attention to the other features of atelectasis allows ready differentiation of this condition. Both congenital hypoplasia of the pulmonary artery and Macleod's syndrome are usually associated with a relatively small lung. The latter condition is now considered to be acquired from an obliterative bronchiolitis in infancy or early childhood. The sequel is a distal obstructive emphysema (which can be demonstrated with an expiratory film) and bronchiectasis in association with a diminution in the pulmonary vasculature.

3. The Solitary Pulmonary Mass

A major problem is posed by the presence, often unexpected, of an intrapulmonary mass on the chest radiograph. The basic difficulty is deciding whether or not the lesion is malignant.

The incidence of malignancy in most large series of solitary pulmonary masses is between 40 and 50 per cent, with an incidence of about 70 per cent in patients older than 50 years of age.

The lesion in question is usually a well circumscribed, intrapulmonary opacity, between 0.5 cm and 6.0 cm in diameter, which is not cavitating and is the only visible abnormality on a chest radiograph. Thus there is no associated hilar or mediastinal adenopathy, no diaphragmatic paralysis, no adjacent bony destruction and no other intrapulmonary opacity. Some causes of such a lesion are listed in Table 3.1.

Bronchial carcinoma, metastasis, abscess, granuloma, and hamartoma account for most solitary

Table 3.1. Some causes of a solitary pulmonary mass.

Bronchial carcinoma
Metastasis
Bronchial adenoma
Hamartoma
Granuloma
Abscess
Arteriovenous malformation
Pulmonary varix
Hydatid cyst
Bronchial cyst
Sequestration
Pulmonary infarct
Haematoma
Bronchocoele
Rheumatoid nodule
Wegener's granuloma

pulmonary masses in the UK. Most granulomas in the UK are tuberculous. Histoplasmosis and coccidioidomycosis are common in parts of the USA and Canada. All the lesions listed may produce an identical appearance on the films. In differentiating them attention should be paid to the following points:

1. Authenticity of the lesion.
2. Age and sex of the patient.
3. Relevant clinical history.
4. Presence or absence on previous films.

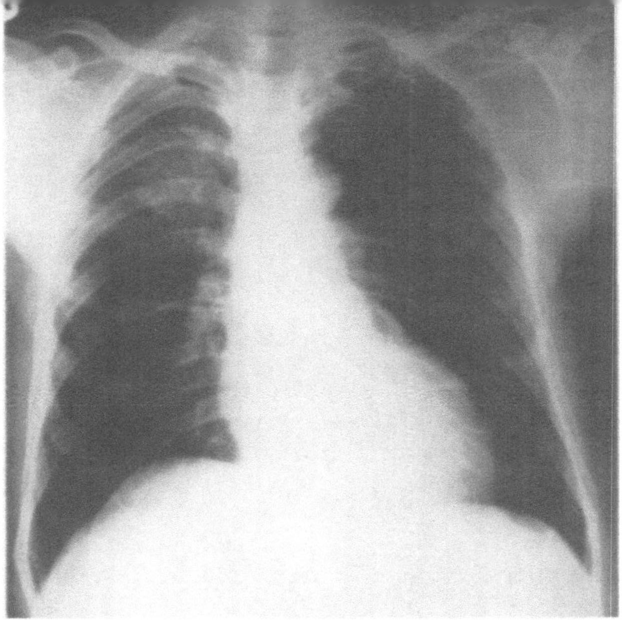

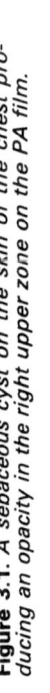

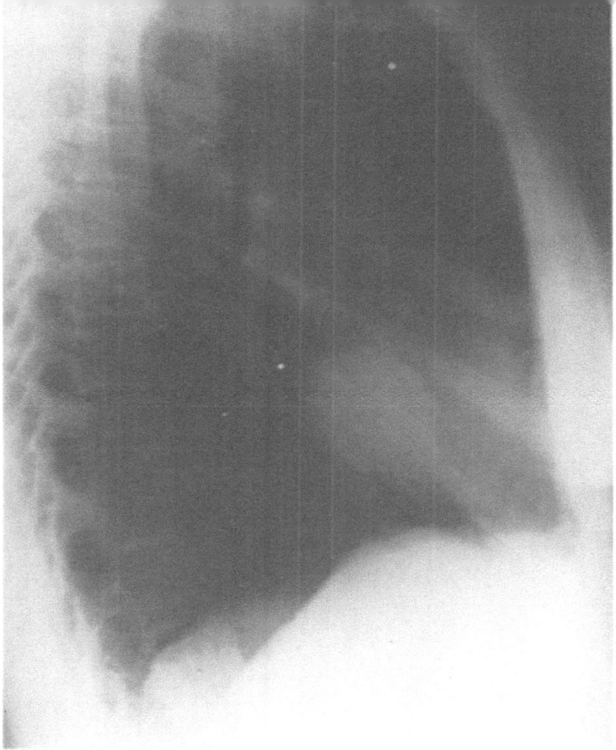

Figure 3.1. A sebaceous cyst on the skin of the chest producing an opacity in the right upper zone on the PA film.

Figure 3.2. Encysted pleural fluid. Note the slightly elliptical configuration and the situation along the line of the oblique fissure.

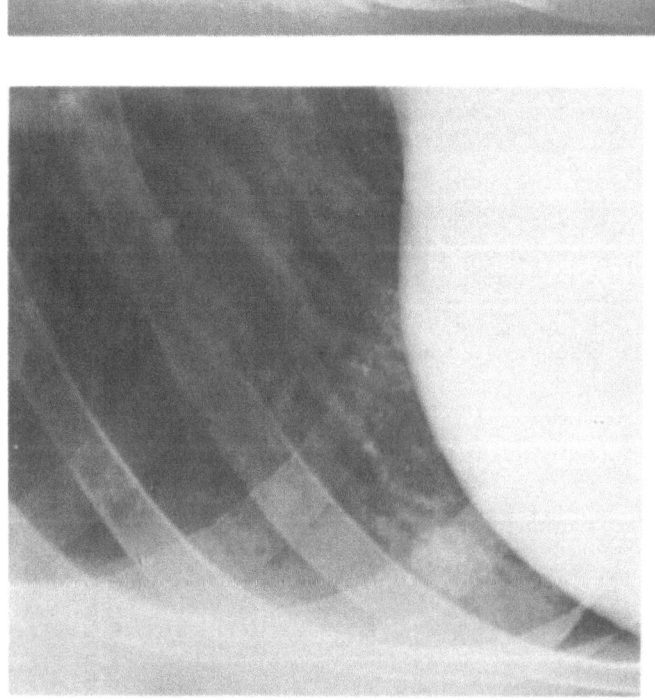

Figure 3.3. (a and b) Healing rib fracture, anterior aspect right seventh rib, differentiated from an intrapulmonary lesion by the coned oblique view.

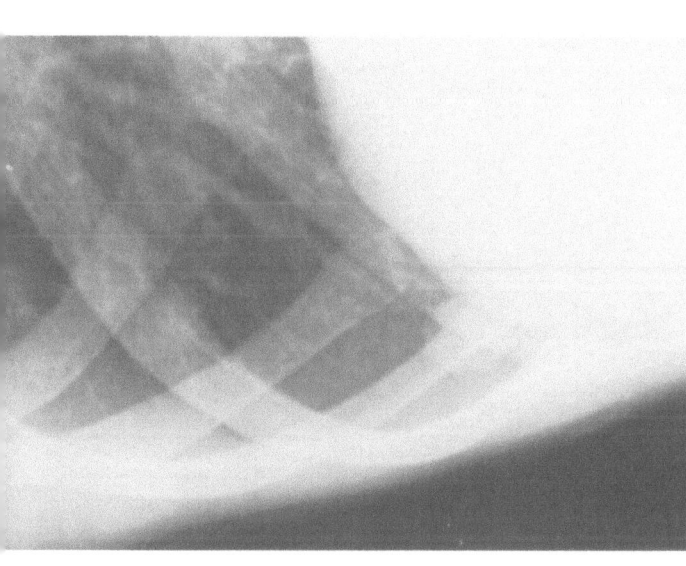

Figure 3.4. *Solitary intrapulmonary metastasis from a renal carcinoma. Note the similarity with Figure 3.3a.*

5. Tomography — presence of calcium.
   margins of lesion.
   feeding or draining vessels.

6. Variation in size with respiration.

Artefacts, such as hair plaits, and cutaneous structures, such as melanomas, nipples and sebaceous cysts (Figure 3.1) may simulate an intrapulmonary abnormality. Interlobar effusions may also cause problems in diagnosis (Figure 3.2). Overinvestigation occasionally occurs in such cases and is highly embarrassing. It is more difficult to differentiate some chest wall and pleural tumours, but by careful attention to their radiographic appearances, and with the aid of oblique films and fluoroscopy, this can often be achieved (Figures 3.3 and 3.4).

Bronchial carcinomas are rare in patients younger than 40 years of age, and such benign lesions as hamartomas, granulomas and congenital abnormalities (AV malformation; bronchial cysts) should be considered in the diagnosis.

If the patient has, or has had a primary malignant neoplasm, the lesion should be considered as metastatic (Figure 3.4). Hydatid disease is endemic in some countries and common with certain occupations (Figure 3.5). A recent history of chest trauma should suggest the possibility of a pulmonary haematoma (Figure 3.6), while an intrapulmonary rheumatoid

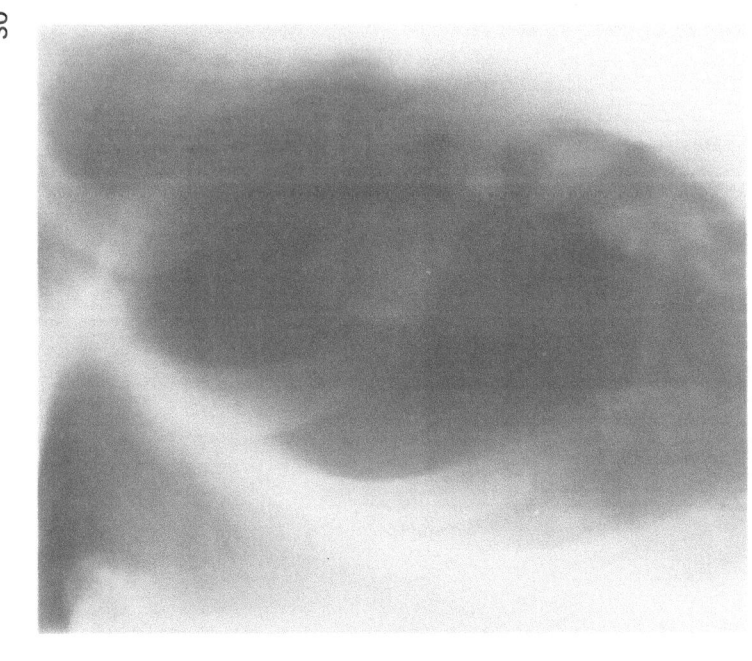

Figure 3.5. *Hydatid cyst (courtesy of Dr D. Gregg). Compare with Figure 3.2.*

Figure 3.6. *Intrapulmonary haematoma. This film was taken following a haemoptysis five days after blunt trauma to the chest.*

nodule is unusual without rheumatoid arthritis. A resolving pulmonary infarct can prove particularly difficult without serial films (Figure 3.7).

It is essential to obtain previous films if such are available. A lesion which has not changed in size or appearance over two years is almost always benign.

Tomography

Tomography allows better definition of a lesion than plain radiography. Much has been written about differentiating benign and malignant lesions on the basis of the margins of the mass. It is now accepted that this is unreliable. Very smooth, well defined lesions are usually, but not necessarily, benign (Figure 3.8). The converse is not true; lesions with irregular, ill defined or spiculated margins may be malignant or benign (Figure 3.9).

Tomography is of more importance in demonstrating calcifications within a mass (Figure 3.10). Tuberculomas account for most calcified intrapulmonary masses in the UK (Figure 3.11); here the calcium is usually in the form of a central nidus or is laminar. A minority (probably less than 10 per cent) of hamartomas have a mass of craggy central calcifications – eponymously called 'popcorn'. Vascular malformations very rarely calcify. In any event, calcification almost invariably indicates that the lesion is benign.

31

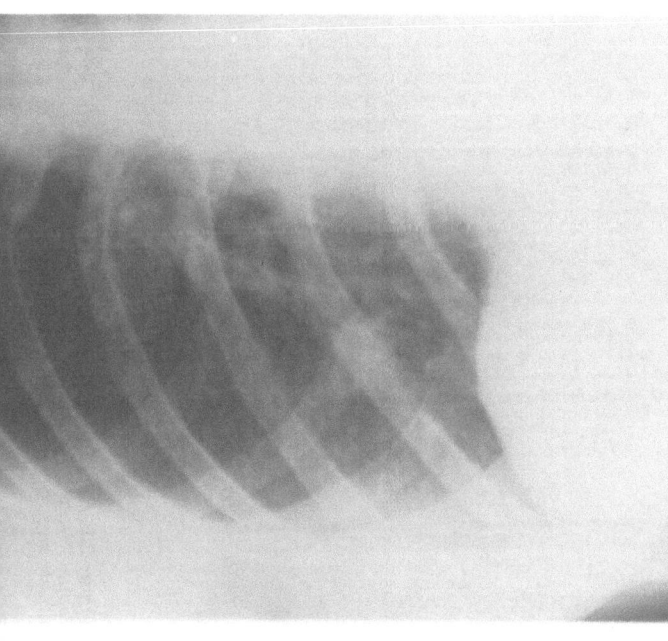

Figure 3.7. Resolving pulmonary infarct, right lower lobe. This lesion had completely disappeared four weeks later.

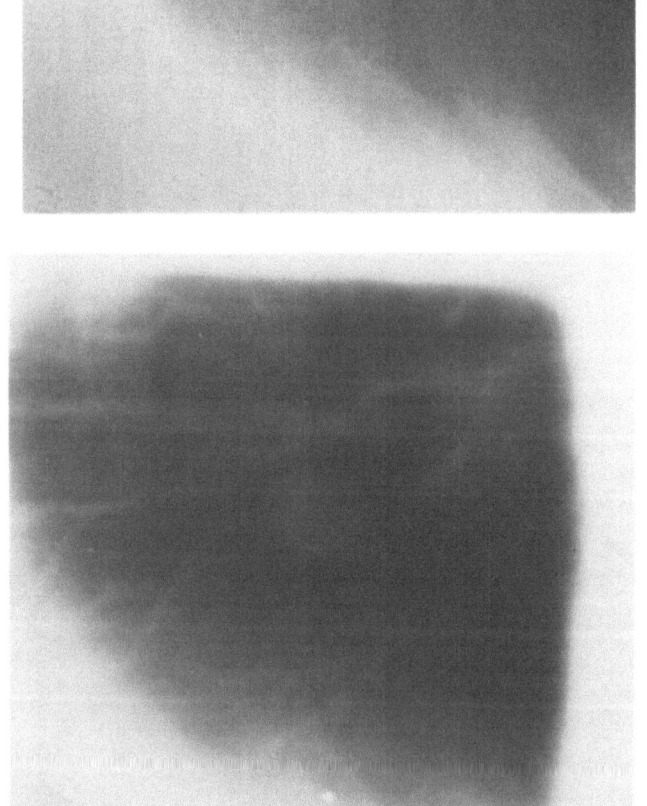

Figure 3.8. Hamartoma. Diagnosis was established by needle biopsy. Note the very well defined smooth outline, which is highly suggestive of a benign lesion.

Figure 3.9. Bronchial carcinoma, clearly defined by tomography. Note the irregular margin, which is in keeping with, although not diagnostic of, a malignant lesion. Diagnosis was established by needle biopsy.

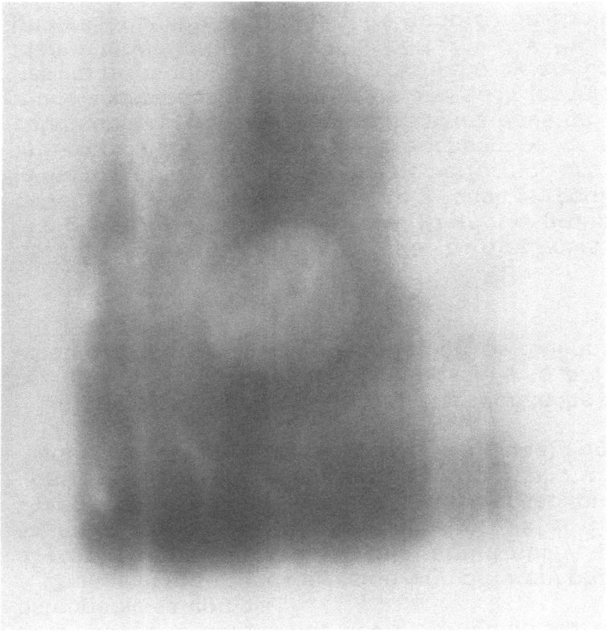

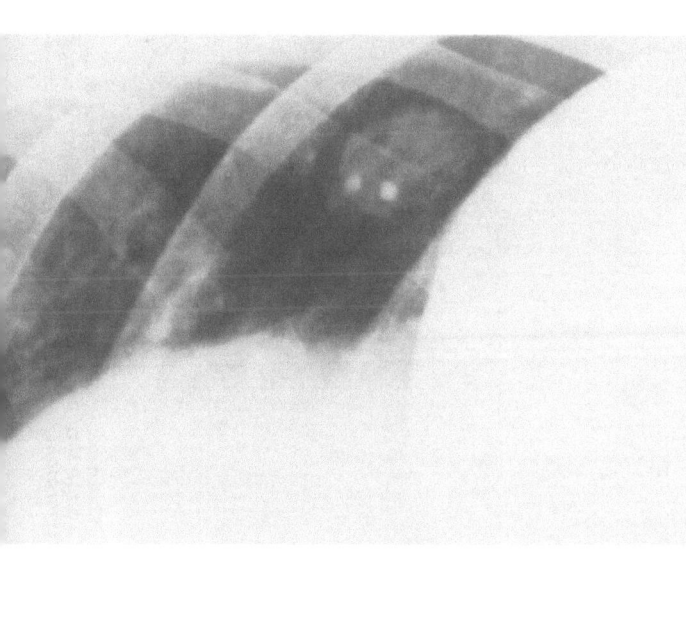

Figure 3.10. Calcification within a solitary metastasis from a osteogenic sarcoma. This is one of the few metastases which can calcify.

Figure 3.11. Tuberculoma containing small nodules of calcification.

Figure 3.12. *Arteriovenous malformation. A lateral tomogram reveals a large draining vessel (arrowed) which is diagnostic of the abnormality.*

There are two exceptions to this rule: eccentrically situated calcification, which may indicate a tuberculous scar with an adjacent carcinoma, and the calcification and bone sometimes seen in metastases from osteogenic sarcomas.

Change in the size of the lesion with different phases of respiration suggests a vascular abnormality, such as an arteriovenous malformation or varix. Such changes are difficult to elicit, and vascular malformations are better demonstrated by tomography when feeding or draining vessels may be seen (Figure 3.12).

Unfortunately, even after paying attention to the preceding points, it is frequently impossible to predict whether a particular lesion is benign or malignant.

Biopsy

Sputum cytology may provide a diagnosis of malignancy, but the yield is low. There is a group of patients in whom a more direct approach is required in the form of a biopsy. This can be performed using a thoracotomy, via the flexible bronchoscope or percutaneously. The latter two approaches have gained much acceptance in recent years and each technique has its protagonists. In good practice they are complementary. Both are usually performed without a general anaesthetic, and require good cytopathology facilities and the use of image intensification. Needle biopsy is quick to perform (15 to 20 minutes) and is a good way of establishing whether or not a mass is malignant (about 85 per cent of malignant lesions will be correctly diagnosed). Approximately 20 per cent of patients develop a pneumothorax. Haemoptysis is infrequent and usually insignificant, but is a potentially serious complication. It is particularly likely to occur in immunosuppressed patients and if vascular masses are biopsied.

Although peripheral pulmonary masses are seldom visible through the flexible bronchoscope, this instrument permits the passage of fine biopsy forceps and brushes which can be directed into the lesion, preferably under fluoroscopic control. The positive yield in malignant lesions is not quite as high as with needle biopsy. A pneumothorax is a rare complication, and haemorrhage is seldom severe and is readily controlled. The procedure takes approximately 45 minutes.

Before either of these two methods of biopsy is performed, it is important to be sure whether the answer obtained will alter the management of the patient. This usually means obviating the need for a thoracotomy.

4. Pulmonary Collapse

Collapse, or atelectasis, implies a loss of volume of the whole or part of the lung. The most important cause of such a loss of volume is partial or complete occlusion of a lobar or segmental bronchus. This form of collapse is a common and important feature of serious underlying disease. Its early recognition is imperative if the underlying abnormality is to be dealt with and if complete re-expansion of the atelectatic lung is to be achieved. The causes of such obstruction are multiple and diverse. The most important are listed in Table 4.1.

Table 4.1. Causes of bronchial obstruction.

Bronchial carcinoma
Bronchial adenoma
Other tumours (e.g. Hodgkin's disease)
Enlarged lymph nodes
Tuberculous bronchostenosis
Inhaled foreign body
Mucous plugs

Obstruction of the airway results in resorption of gas distally. The degree of collapse depends upon the degree and duration of obstruction and on the underlying state of the lung. Thus, the collapse following the inhalation of a foreign body is usually immediate and considerable in degree, unlike that seen distal to a carcinoma or bronchial adenoma where the changes occur more slowly and where the degree of collapse may be less because of an associated pneumonia with consolidation.

The obstruction of a segmental bronchus often fails to result in collapse. This is because the pores of Kohn and canals of Lambert allow communication and 'collateral air drift' between the alveoli or bronchioli of one segment and those adjacent. No such collateral ventilation occurs between lobes, as they are bounded by pleural surfaces, and lobar collapse is not prevented by this mechanism.

It can now be appreciated that collapse is a common, but not inevitable, result of bronchial obstruction. Conversely collapse may occur without major bronchial occlusion, for example, the loss of volume which sometimes accompanies a severe 'simple' pneumonia (Figure 4.1), and the collapse–consolidation not infrequently found after major chest trauma, where respiration is often inadequate. In the latter situation, bronchiolar mucous plugging and surfactant loss may be causative factors. In this, and in the loss of volume accompanying some 'simple' pneumonias, the patency of the major bronchi is apparent on good quality films or tomograms. As might be anticipated, bronchoscopy is often not particularly helpful in these cases.

Thick horizontal line shadows are often seen in the lower lobes of severely ill patients. They are quite common after major abdominal surgery, myocardial infarction and severe trauma. They are also a feature of pulmonary thromboembolism. They are thought to represent subsegmental areas of collapse, and are known as linear or plate atelectasis. Their aetiology is uncertain.

Another form of atelectasis is so-called passive atelectasis. Anything which increases the pleural pressure displaces the adjacent lung, which will also tend to reduce in volume. Thus a pneumothorax, pleural effusion or thoracoplasty will cause partial collapse of the adjacent lobe or lung. Loss of lung volume also occurs in a variety of fibrotic or destructive pulmonary conditions which result in decreased pulmonary compliance. Loss of volume of the lower lobes is a common finding in fibrosing alveolitis; decreased volume of the upper lobes frequently accompanies 'healed' tuberculosis, and lobar or segmental loss of volume is often present to some degree in bronchiectasis.

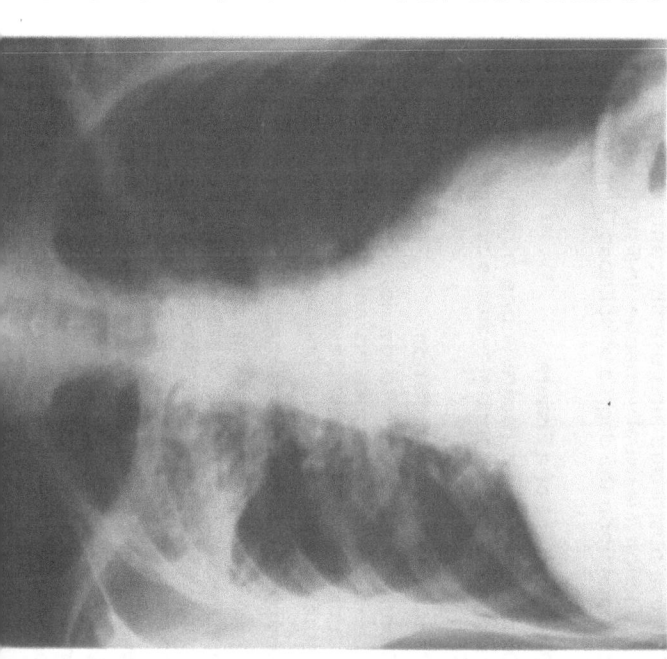

Figure 4.1. *Severe pneumococcal pneumonia causing some loss of volume of the right upper lobe. Note the air-containing bronchi within the lobe.*

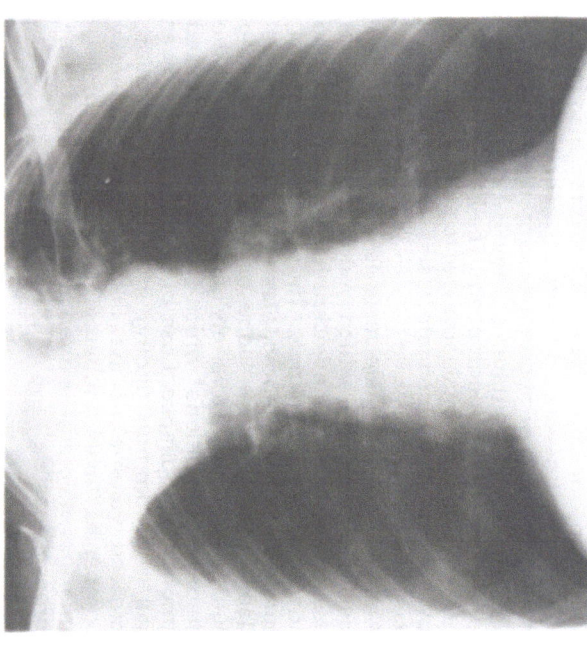

Figure 4.2. *Right upper lobe collapse. The collapsed lobe is homogeneously opaque. The minor fissure has been displaced superomedially.*

Radiographic Signs of Collapse

The Presence of a Radio-opacity

Because obstructed lung usually contains some fluid or infection it is usually opaque: the size of the opacity depends upon the degree of collapse (Figures 4.2 and 4.3).

Displacement of a Fissure

Displacement of a fissure is one of the most readily recognized and important features of collapse (Figure 4.4).

Compensatory Overinflation

Compensatory overinflation is usually most pronounced in younger patients and in collapse of some standing. The most reliable evidence of overinflation is the relative paucity of lung vessels (Figure 4.5).

Upward Displacement of the Diaphragm

Upward displacement of the diaphragm is frequently not present. Of itself it is of little significance and other causes of diaphragmatic displacement should always be remembered.

Mediastinal Displacement

Mediastinal displacement is variable. It is more common in young patients and when there is collapse of one of the larger lobes (for example, left upper lobe).

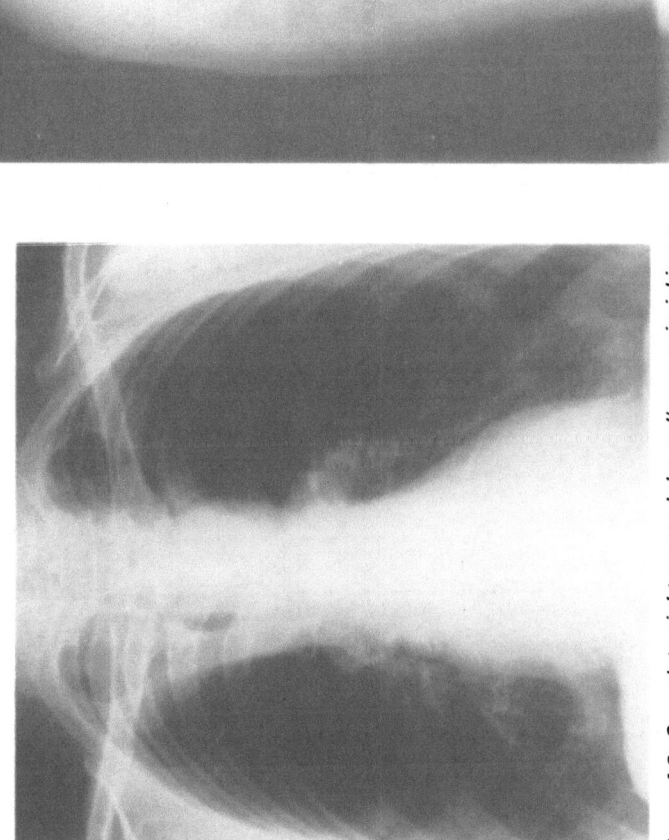

Figure 4.3. Complete right upper lobe collapse mimicking a widened superior mediastinum. The arrow indicates the displaced minor fissure.

Figure 4.4. The lateral film reveals anterior displacement of the left oblique fissure.

Hilar Displacement

Hilar displacement is occasionally pronounced with marked collapse. It is important to recognize more subtle abnormalities, such as both hila at the same level in early lower lobe collapse (Figures 4.6 and 4.7).

Approximation of the Ribs

Approximation of the ribs only occurs when other features already present allow one to make the diagnosis.

The Absence of an Air Bronchogram

The airways distal to an obstructed major bronchus are usually fluid filled. The obstructed lobe therefore usually appears homogeneously opaque, in contrast to a lobar pneumonia where the patent bronchi produce an 'air-bronchogram' (see Figure 4.1).

Upper Lobe Collapse

Each lobe collapses in a characteristic fashion. The classic appearance of right upper lobe collapse is illustrated in Figure 4.2. The PA film is of most value in making the diagnosis. The completely collapsed lobe lies adjacent to the mediastinum and may mimic widening of that structure (Figure 4.3).

The absence of a minor fissure in the left lung

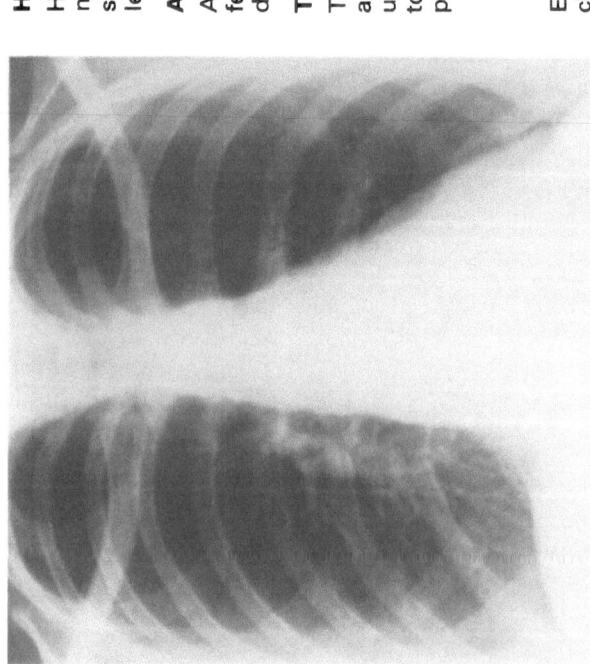

Figure 4.5. *Left lower lobe collapse. The left hilum has been displaced downwards and is almost invisible. The oblique fissure, seen through the heart shadow, outlines the collapsed lobe. Note the paucity of vessels on the left due to compensatory overinflation of the left upper lobe.*

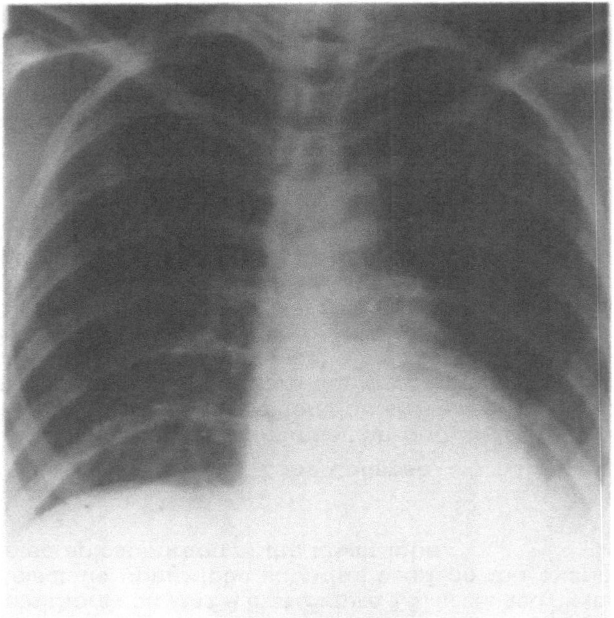

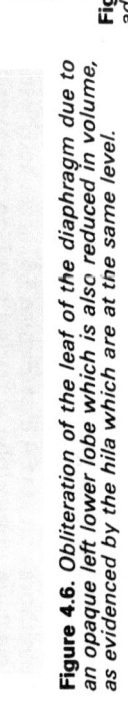

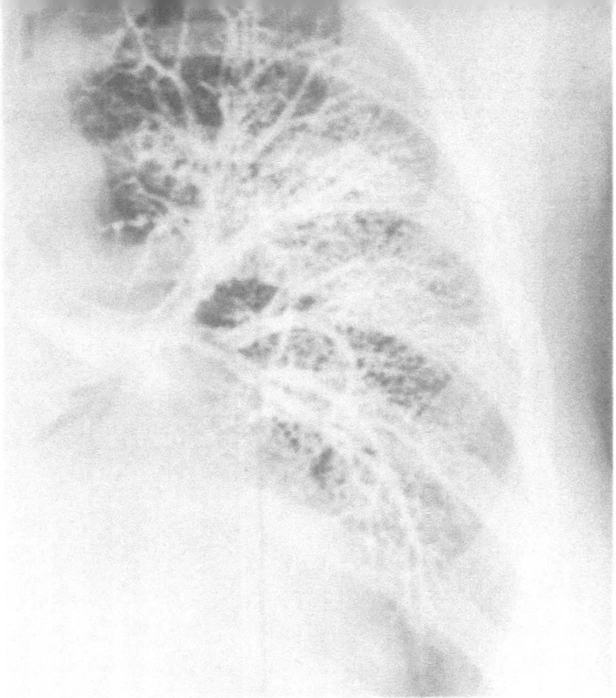

Figure 4.7. A bronchogram reveals a tumour (bronchial adenoma) partially occluding the left lower lobe bronchus.

Figure 4.6. Obliteration of the leaf of the diaphragm due to an opaque left lower lobe which is also reduced in volume, as evidenced by the hila which are at the same level.

41

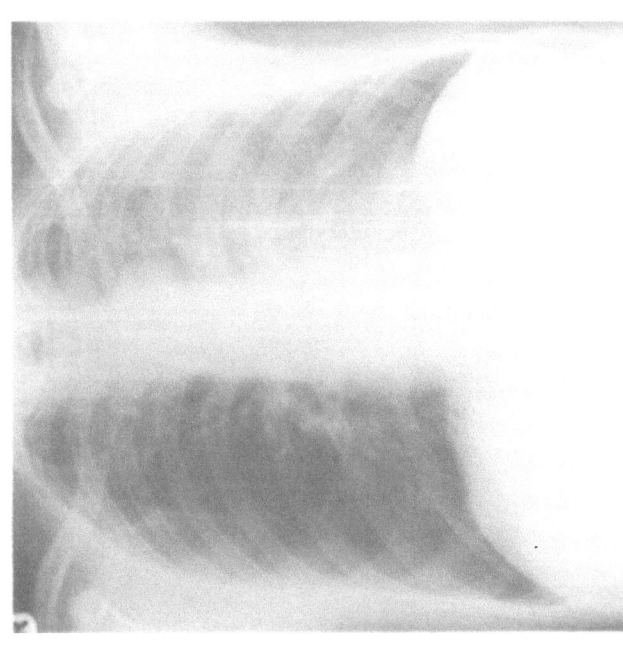

explains the quite different appearance of left upper lobe collapse (Figures 4.4 and 4.8). This lobe collapses both superomedially and anteriorly. The lateral film is invaluable in confirming the diagnosis. The hazy upper hemithorax on the PA film (Figure 4.8) is caused by the atelectatic upper lobe superimposed on the overinflated apical portion of the lower lobe.

Lower Lobe Collapse

Lower lobe collapse is similar on both sides. Asymmetry of the hila and obliteration of the medial aspect of the hemidiaphragm are the most notable features on the PA film (Figure 4.9). The displaced oblique fissure is not always seen on the lateral film because it is frequently also partially rotated and no longer lies tangential to the X-ray beam. Sometimes it is seen on the PA film (Figure 4.5). Oblique views are helpful in elucidating difficult cases.

Middle Lobe Collapse

Right middle lobe collapse is most readily appreciated on the lateral film as a thin, wedge-shaped opacity between the approximated minor and major fissures. It may be suspected on the PA view, where the right heart border is partially obliterated or ill defined —

Figure 4.8. *Left upper lobe collapse producing characteristic hazy left hemithorax. (Compare with right upper lobe collapse in Figure 4.2.)*

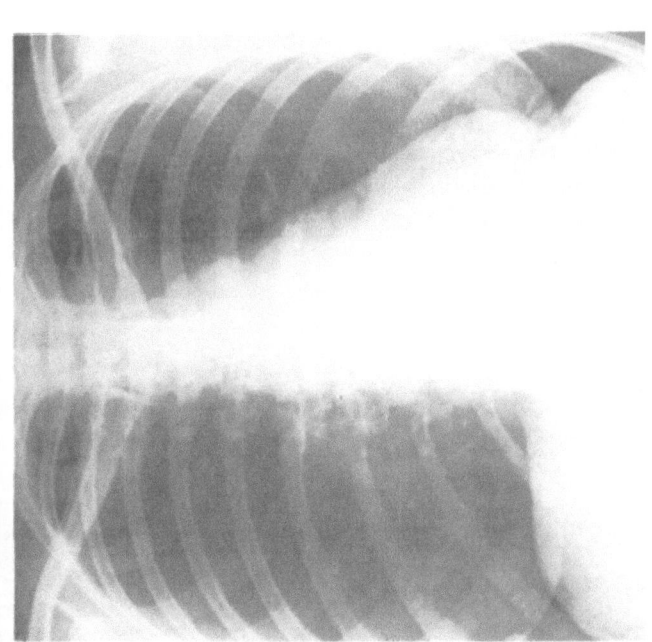

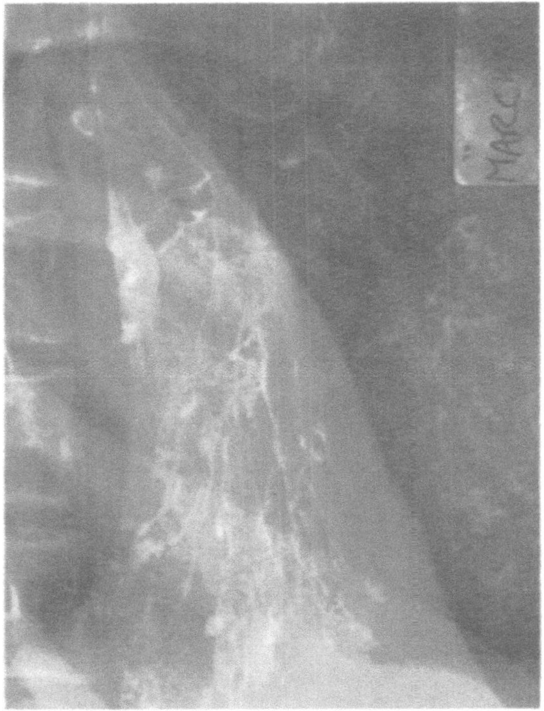

Figure 4.9. (a) Collapse of the left lower lobe on the PA film, (b) A bronchogram reveals crowding of the lower lobe bronchi which are bronchiectatic. The lower lobe bronchus is patent.

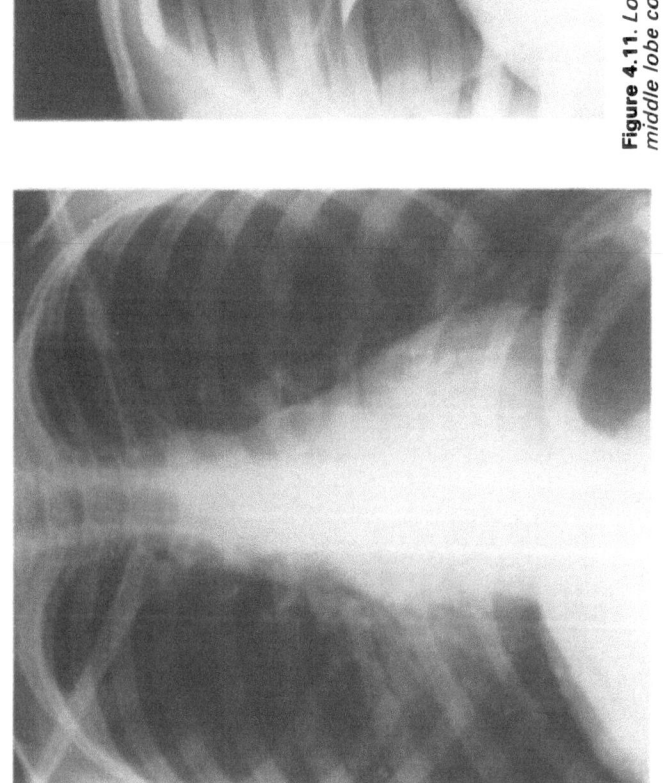

Figure 4.10. Right middle lobe collapse. The only abnormality is a hazy opacity adjacent to and obliterating the right heart border.

Figure 4.11. Lordotic projection establishes the diagnosis of middle lobe collapse.

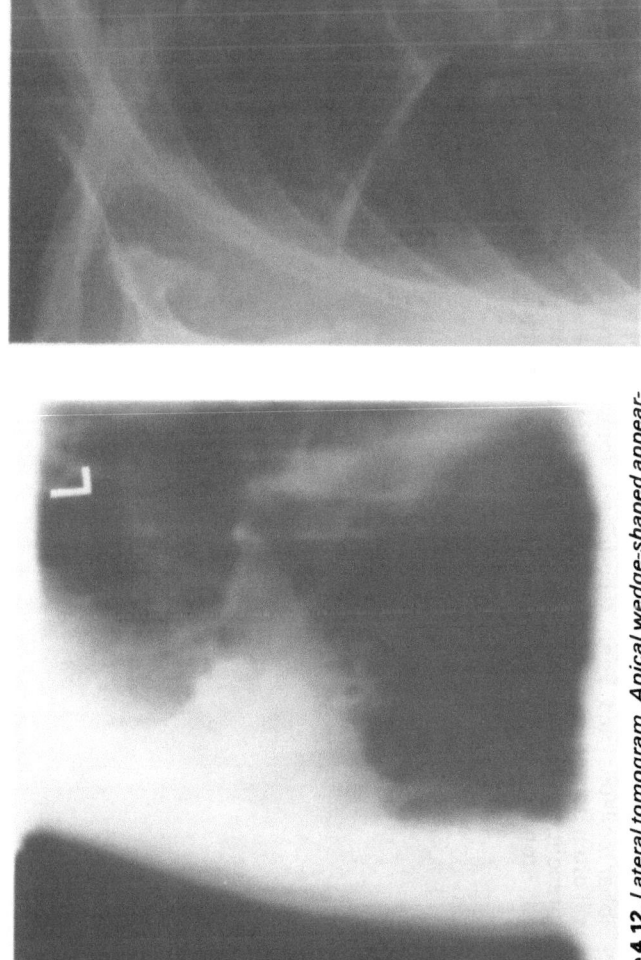

Figure 4.12. Lateral tomogram. Apical wedge-shaped appearance of partial segmental collapse caused by a carcinoma at the origin of the apical segmental bronchus of the lower lobe.

Figure 4.13. Complete collapse of the anterior segment of the right upper lobe producing a thick linear shadow adjacent to the elevated minor fissure (bronchial carcinoma).

45

the 'silhouette sign' (Figure 4.10). Lordotic views and tomography in the lateral position are useful confirmatory techniques (Figure 4.11).

Once lobar collapse has been recognized, tomography will often demonstrate whether an obstructing lesion is present, but bronchoscopy should always be performed. Bronchoscopy allows a complete assessment of the bronchial tree with a tissue diagnosis. Segmental collapse may also be indicative of an underlying tumour. It is more difficult to recognize because there is little, if any, displacement of the normal structures. It produces a wedge-shaped or tubular density, an appearance which is unusual in pneumonia and with which it should obviously not be confused (Figures 4.12 and 4.13).

5. Cavitating Pulmonary Lesions

A pulmonary cavity is represented on the chest radiograph as an opacity within which is an area of radiolucency. When the rim of the cavity is thin, the descriptive term 'ring shadow' is sometimes applied. While cavities are often obvious on standard films, a fluid level is occasionally the only, and all-important, clue to the presence of cavitation. This will obviously not be present on films taken with a vertical beam. This should be remembered when viewing tomographic cuts which have been obtained in the supine position. Overlapping vascular and bony shadows may mimic a cavity. Fluoroscopy, oblique or lordotic views will usually resolve any such problem, but tomography may be required. In addition to providing confirmation that a cavity is present, it allows better definition of the lesion and is frequently employed as an aid to differential diagnosis (Figures 5.1 and 5.2).

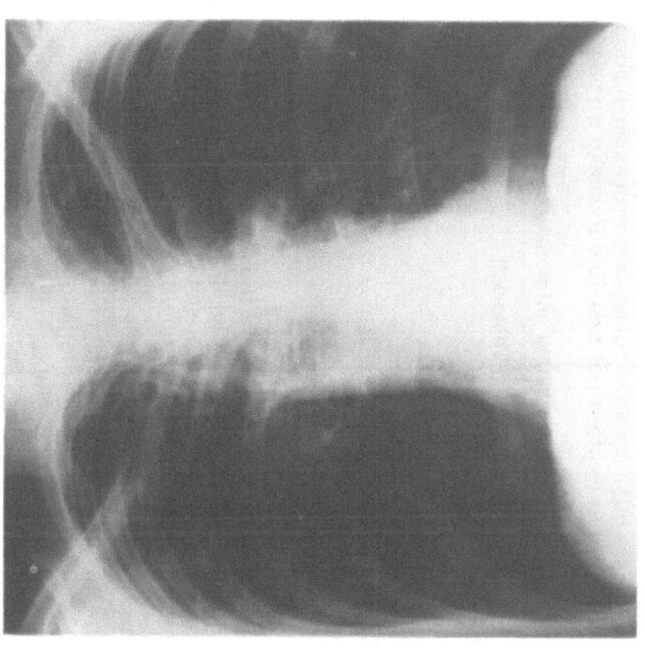

Figure 5.1. *Scarring with loss of volume, right upper lobe, as shown by tracheal shift and an elevated right hilum in a patient with known tuberculosis. There is no obvious cavity.*

47

The Solitary Cavity

The causes of a solitary pulmonary cavity are given in Table 5.1. The clinical state sometimes suggests the diagnosis, but a cavity is not uncommon as an incidental finding. It is often not possible to make a specific

Table 5.1. Causes of a solitary pulmonary cavity.

Cavitating pneumonia (see Table 5.2)
Bronchial carcinoma
Metastatic carcinoma
Hodgkin's lymphoma
Pulmonary infarct
Wegener's granuloma
Rheumatoid nodule
Post-traumatic haematoma
Hydatid cyst
Progressive massive fibrosis

aetiological diagnosis from the films, but a careful appraisal of certain radiographic features and an awareness of the clinical possibilities should assist in the management of the patient.

Position of the Lesion

The position of the lesion is of some importance; it is extremely rare for a tuberculous cavity to be in the anterior aspect of the lung. The apical segments of the upper and lower lobes are favoured sites (Figure 5.2).

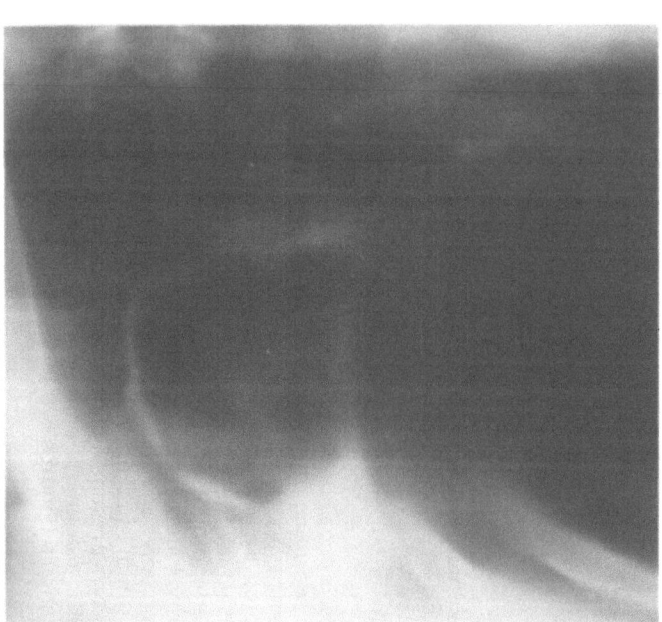

Figure 5.2. A tomogram of the right upper lobe in the same patient as Figure 5.1 reveals a large thin-walled cavity.

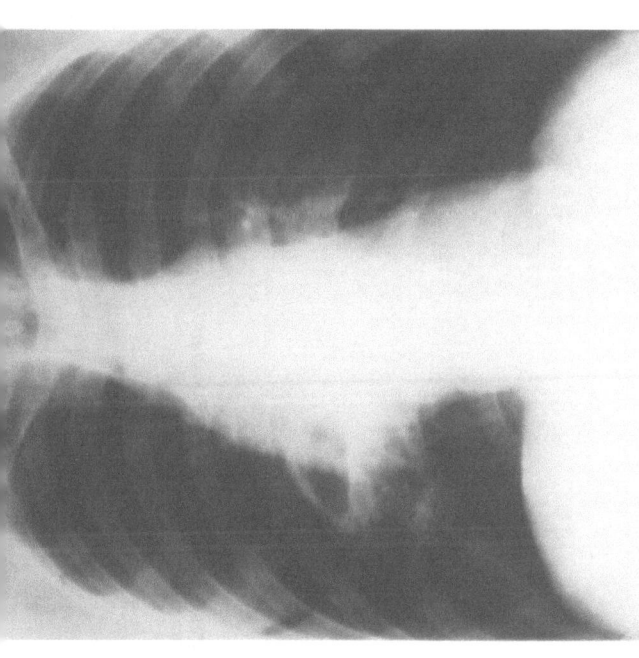

Figure 5.3. *Abscess cavity in the apical segment of the right lower lobe due to aspiration from a dilated oesophagus (achalasia). The latter is responsible for the widened mediastinum and fluid level (arrowed).*

Supraclavicular cavitation is more likely to be caused by tuberculosis than anything else. Chronic allergic alveolitis, sarcoidosis, bronchopulmonary aspergillosis and ankylosing spondylitis are less common causes of scarred upper lobes with or without cavitation. Most abscesses which are secondary to aspiration are situated posteriorly, in the lower lobes (Figure 5.3) or in the axillary region of the upper lobes.

Age

An underlying congenital abnormality, such as a bronchial cyst or sequestration, should come high on the list of possibilities in children and young adults (Figure 5.4). Sequestrated segments are almost invariably situated in the lower lobes and are more common on the left than the right side.

Cavity Wall

The appearance of the wall of the cavity is of some diagnostic value. Most cavitating neoplasms have thick, irregular walls (Figure 5.5), and tuberculous cavities tend to be thin-walled (Figure 5.2). The converse may occur, so cavity wall thickness is an unreliable diagnostic point. When the wall is merely represented by a line shadow, a bulla is most likely. However, staphylococcal pneumatocoeles, post-traumatic 'cysts' and some tuberculous cavities have the same appearance.

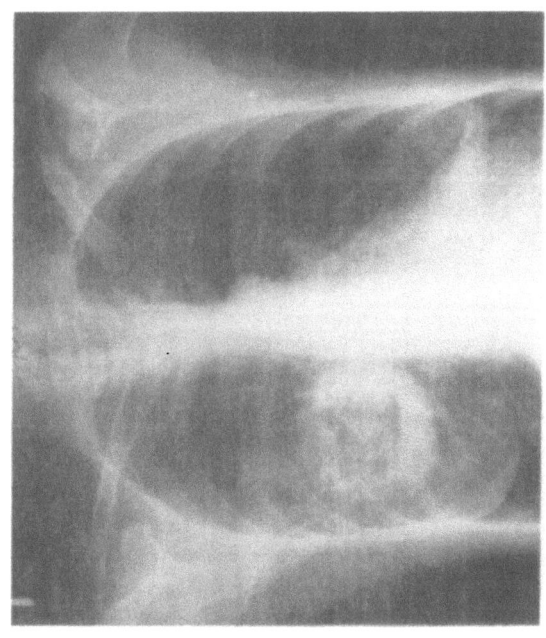

Figure 5.5. *Typical thick-walled cavitating squamous cell bronchial carcinoma.*

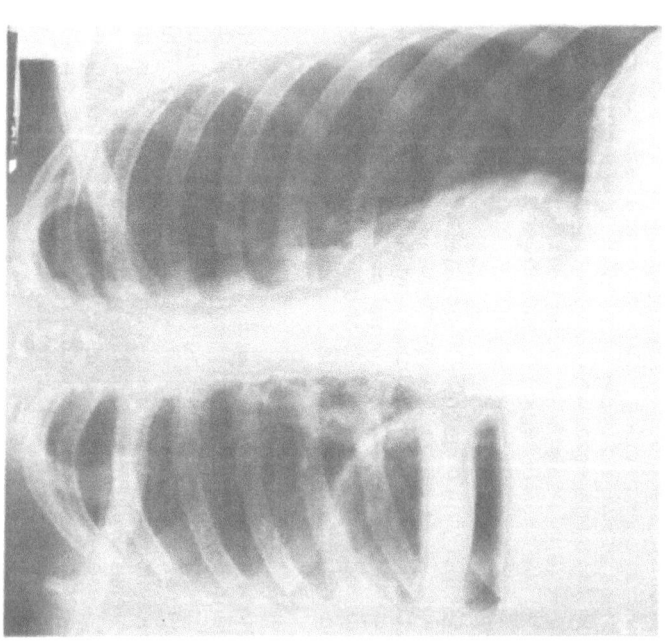

Figure 5.4. *Right lower lobe abscess in an 18-year-old male, caused by an infected bronchial cyst.*

Surrounding Lung

Cavitation may be represented only by a fluid level within a large area of consolidation representing pneumonia. It is then of prime importance to determine whether this is a primary suppurative pneumonia or whether there is an underlying bronchial occlusion (Table 5.2). The latter is usually caused by tumour,

Table 5.2. Cavitating pneumonias.

Primary bacterial pneumonia
 Tuberculous
 Staphylococcal
 Klebsiella
 Pseudomonas
 Non-specific
Underlying bronchial occlusion
 Tumour
 Foreign body
 Bronchostenosis
Aspiration pneumonia
Fungal pneumonia
Underlying pulmonary abnormality
 Bronchiectasis
 Sequestration
 Bronchial cyst

bronchostenosis or foreign body and is frequently associated with some loss of volume in the pulmonary lobe or segments involved. Such bronchial occlusion

can be demonstrated by bronchography, but bronchoscopy usually allows a definitive diagnosis and should be performed with some urgency. Tuberculous cavities are sometimes surrounded by typical, small, ill-defined nodular shadows representing local bronchopneumonic spread (Figure 5.6). Staphylococcal pneumonia is one of the most common primary cavitating pneumonias. A thin-walled 'cyst' or pneumatocoele is the occasional residue (Figure 5.7). In children quite large thin-walled pneumatocoeles may appear quite abruptly and allow a specific diagnosis. Pseudomonas and Klebsiella pneumonias also cavitate (Figure 5.8). The latter occasionally expand the involved lobe. While these are the classical primary cavitating bacterial pneumonias, any pneumonia may cavitate, especially when inadequately treated.

The possibility of a fungal infection should always be considered in any chronic cavitating pneumonia. Actinomycosis may cause adjacent rib destruction. Histoplasmosis and coccidioidomycosis may occur in patients who have lived in North America. Hodgkin's lymphoma, rheumatoid disease, pulmonary infarction and Wegener's granuloma are rare causes of an irregular, thick-walled cavity. They cannot be differentiated from a cavitating carcinoma. An area of progressive massive fibrosis in coalworkers' pneumoconiosis occasionally cavitates, and may be productive of an inky

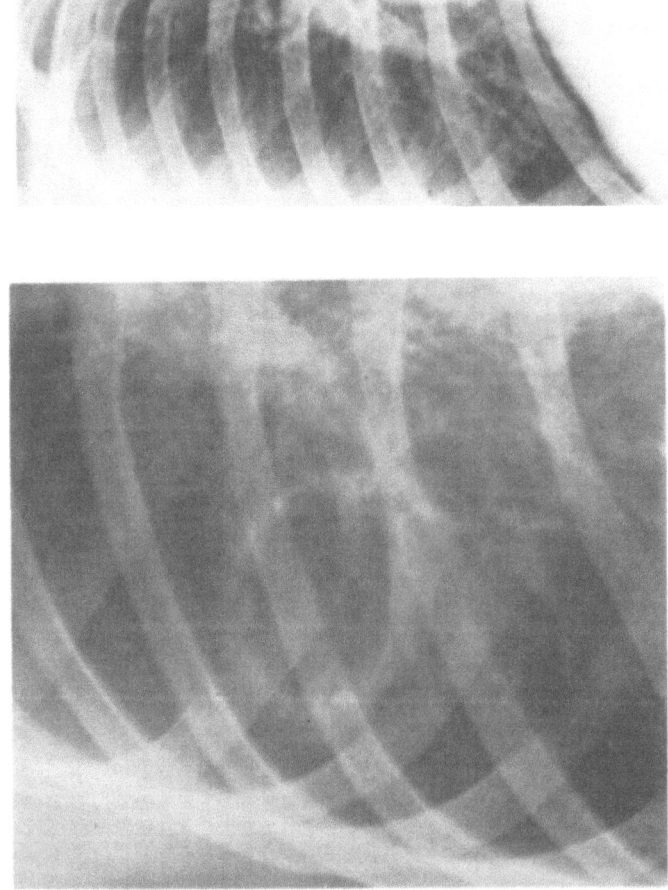

Figure 5.7. *Thin-walled cyst left midzone as a residue of staphylococcal pneumonia.*

Figure 5.6. *Tuberculosis. Cavity in the right lower lobe with typical surrounding bronchopneumonic spread.*

black sputum. There is associated pulmonary shrinkage, and a diffuse nodular pattern can usually be detected throughout the remainder of the lung field.

Contents of the Cavity

Some attention should be paid to the contents of the cavity. The importance of a fluid level in establishing the presence of cavitation has already been mentioned. A mobile soft tissue mass within the cavity is most commonly seen in tuberculous (Figure 5.9) and neoplastic cavities. The same appearance occasionally occurs with ruptured hydatid cysts and cavitating pulmonary haematomas. The intracavitary mass may represent blood or necrotic debris. Old tuberculous cavities may also contain fungus balls (mycetoma) (Figure 5.9). In these instances there is a high level of serum precipitins. An intracavitary calcific density (cavernolith) is a very rare finding, and usually occurs in an old tuberculous cavity with an associated bronchostenosis.

Hilar and Mediastinal Lymphadenopathy

Hilar and mediastinal lymphadenopathy should always be looked for carefully. It is uncommon in primary bacterial pneumonias and in cavitating tuberculosis; it is usually evidence of a bronchial carcinoma. Lymphomas and fungal infections occasionally

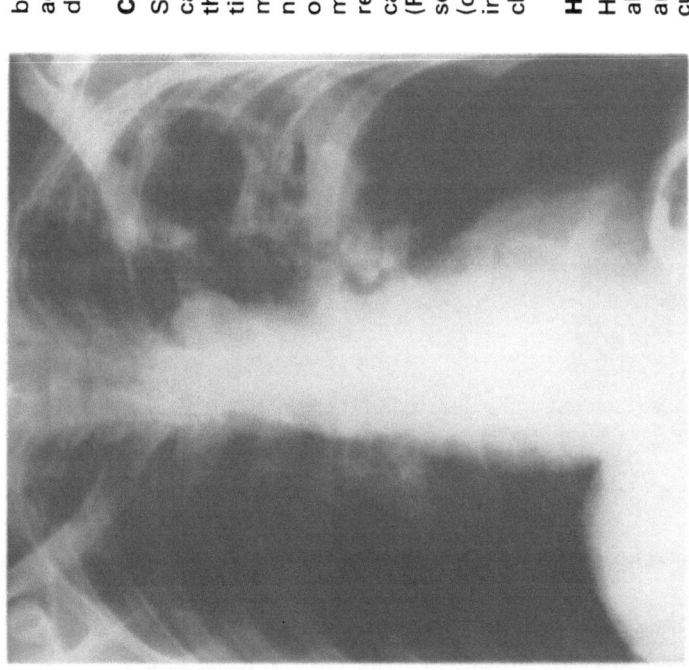

Figure 5.8. *Cavitating Klebsiella pneumonia.*

53

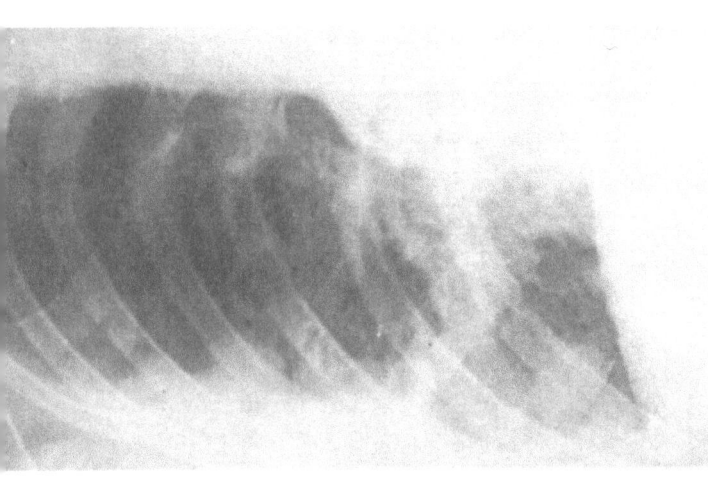

Figure 5.9. *Tuberculous cavity with mycetoma. Note the characteristic halo around the fungus ball within the cavity.*

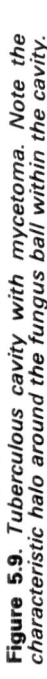

Figure 5.10. *Multiple cavitating opacities in both lungs—pyaemic abscess.*

produce the same appearance. The latter should be borne in mind, particularly with the increasing numbers of immunosuppressed patients.

Other Clues to Malignancy

Phrenic nerve palsy, indicated by a high diaphragm, and bony metastases are other infrequent but important clues to malignancy which can be obtained from the chest radiograph.

Clinical history and findings, together with the examination of the sputum for organisms and cells, may provide the diagnosis. Bronchoscopic examination or percutaneous needle aspiration and biopsy are extremely valuable methods of establishing the diagnosis and should be performed at an early stage in the assessment of the patient.

Multiple Pulmonary Cavities

Multiple pulmonary cavities (Figure 5.10) are unusual: the causes are listed in Table 5.3. The most common causes are septic infarcts and multiple metastases,

Table 5.3. Causes of multiple pulmonary cavities.

Metastases
Pyaemic abscesses
Pulmonary infarcts
Rheumatoid nodules
Wegener's granuloma
Hydatid cysts

which are usually from a primary tumour of squamous origin. The diagnosis is usually obvious from the clinical history.

6. Pulmonary Thromboembolism

Most cases of pulmonary thromboembolism are caused by obstruction of a pulmonary artery by a thrombus dislodged from the veins of the legs, pelvis or abdomen. Rarely, the thrombus may originate in the right atrium and upper limbs.

Pulmonary artery thrombosis may supervene upon, and is occasionally the primary cause of, pulmonary artery occlusion. Other forms of pulmonary embolism (caused by tumour, fat, etc.) will not be considered here. Evidence of pulmonary thromboembolism is found in about 15 per cent of necropsies performed on adults dying in hospitals. In three to five per cent of hospital deaths pulmonary thromboembolism is the principal cause of death, and in 50 per cent of these cases there is evidence of previous embolism or infarction. The necessity for an accurate means of diagnosis is, therefore, apparent. It is important to realise that

pulmonary thromboembolism does not imply the presence of pulmonary infarction. This occurs in only a small proportion, perhaps 15 per cent, of embolic episodes.

Unfortunately, the disease is a great dissembler, and a fundamental and important prerequisite for early and accurate diagnosis is a high index of suspicion on the parts of the clinician and radiologist. The radiological features depend largely upon the size and number of emboli, their site of impaction and the presence or absence of associated pulmonary infarction. Therefore it is preferable, for discussion purposes and from a practical point of view, to differentiate between pulmonary embolism with and without infarction, and also between the various forms of embolism, which fall broadly into three main groups:

1. Massive pulmonary embolism.

2. Embolism of lobar or segmental arteries.

3. Multiple small peripheral emboli.

Massive Pulmonary Embolism

Massive pulmonary embolism occurs when there is embolism of the main pulmonary artery or its two major branches. It implies involvement of at least 50 per cent of the vascular tree. The clinical features are usually dramatic and well known (sudden collapse, dyspnoea, with central chest pain) and the condition constitutes a medical emergency. A plain chest radiograph is often normal. Careful appraisal of the film may, however, reveal hyperlucent areas caused by a paucity of vessels indicating areas of pulmonary oligaemia. Good quality radiographs are obviously essential. The main pulmonary artery is sometimes enlarged and the hilar shadows may appear plump (probably because of a combination of clot within the artery and its fairly abrupt termination related to peripheral underfilling). Infarct shadows, if present, usually indicate a previous embolic episode. Acute pulmonary oedema occasionally occurs.

The suspected diagnosis can be confirmed by pulmonary angiography. In a well-equipped centre this takes relatively little time. Screening facilities with image intensification are required and equipment for cardiac monitoring and resuscitation is mandatory. The catheter, introduced via an antecubital vein, is ideally placed with its tip in the main pulmonary artery; failing this, a right atrial injection will usually suffice. Selective injections are sometimes required and they improve diagnostic accuracy. The embolus is seen as a filling defect within the artery (Figures 6.1 and 6.2). This examination allows confirmation of the suspected diagnosis, permits pressure recordings to be obtained

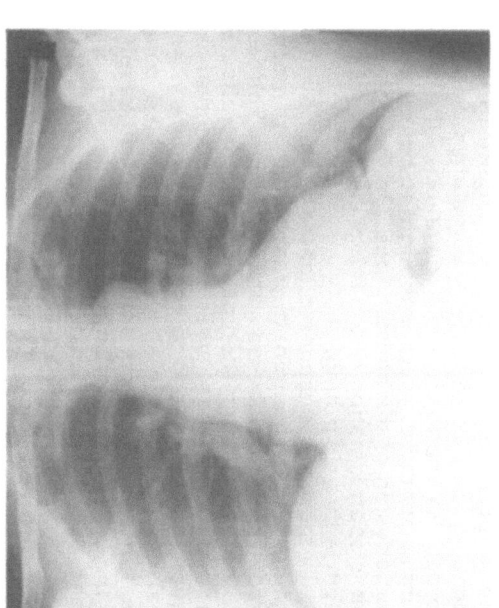

Figure 6.1. *Clear lungs in a patient suspected of having a massive pulmonary embolus. (Scapular shadows overly the lateral lung fields.)*

and provides the surgeon with the necessary information before surgery or a line for streptokinase infusion, depending upon the method of treatment.

Where these facilities are not available and when

Embolism of Lobar or Segmental Arteries— Without Infarction

Embolism of the lobar or segmental arteries is a much more common condition than massive pulmonary embolism. The clinical features are notoriously fickle and it is in this group that the diagnosis is most likely to be missed.

The plain chest radiograph is frequently normal. Rarely there may be oligaemic areas in the distribution of the lobes or segments involved (Figure 6.3). The descending pulmonary artery sometimes appears engorged. An important sign is elevation of the relevant hemidiaphragm, which is thought to be related to underperfusion of the affected lobe. On the right the result is approximation of the minor fissure and diaphragm with a clear lung.

Ideally these cases are investigated further by lung scanning, using albumin microspheres or macroaggregates, usually labelled with technetium. The scan reveals areas of diminished perfusion in the affected areas (Figure 6.4). These areas follow a segmental distribution, usually extend to the lung periphery, and sometimes possess the shape of a truncated cone. Several perfusion defects are often seen, in keeping with the belief that most emboli are multiple (Figures 6.4 and 6.5). Anterior, posterior, oblique and lateral views are usually obtained. Correlation with the plain chest radiograph is imperative. The perfusion scan is

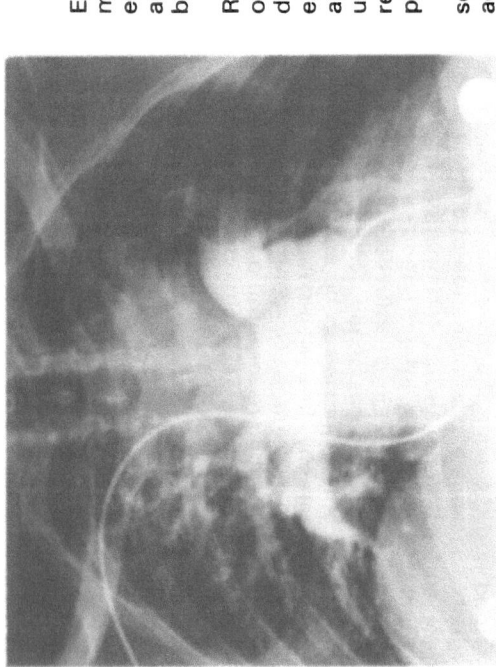

Figure 6.2. *Pulmonary angiogram immediately after Figure 6.1. was taken, showing an embolus occluding the left main pulmonary artery.*

surgery is not contemplated, lung scanning may be performed to advantage. The gamma camera, which allows a rapid examination with multiple views, is preferable to rectilinear scanning devices.

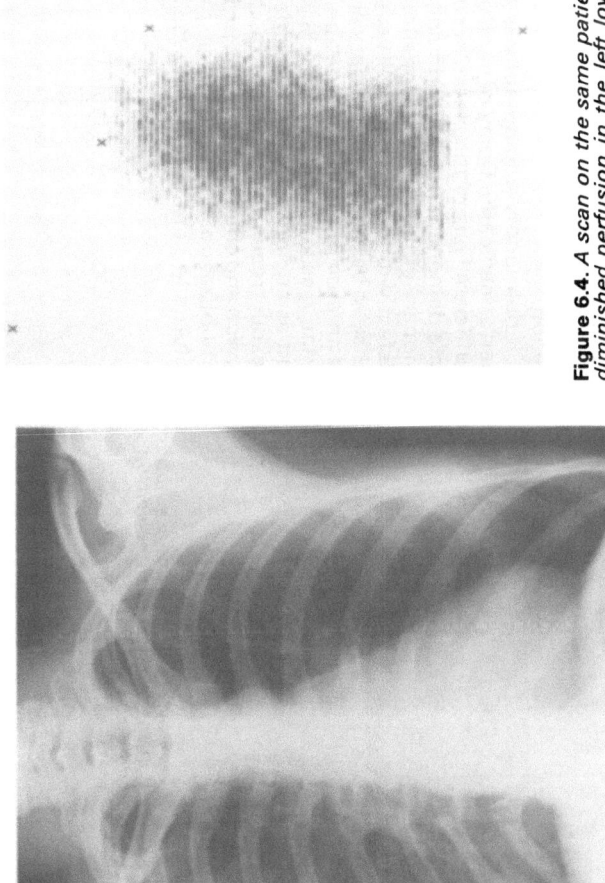

Figure 6.3. A 32-year-old female with abrupt onset of tachypnoea and dyspnoea. There is a hyperlucent area on the left lower zone. The appearances are otherwise normal.

Figure 6.4. A scan on the same patient as Figure 6.3 reveals diminished perfusion in the left lower lobe. The scan was normal four weeks later.

a sensitive but non-specific indicator of embolism. Any pulmonary or pleural opacity will produce a 'positive' scan as will obstructive airways disease. However a normal perfusion scan virtually excludes a recent embolism. The limitations of the perfusion scan have been largely overcome and the specificity greatly improved by the use of combined ventilation scans using xenon.

If pulmonary angiography is required, it should be performed early. Delay of even a day or so may permit sufficient lysis of the clot to occur to preclude an accurate demonstration of its presence. As in massive pulmonary embolism, the clot should be seen as a filling defect within the opacified vessel for a definite diagnosis to be made. A secondary and non-specific feature is an area of diminished perfusion.

Lung scanning is less expensive and not as unpleasant as angiography for the patient. Because it may be readily repeated, progress of the lesion may be followed and changing patterns provide evidence of fresh embolization. In most cases pulmonary blood flow returns to normal after six weeks to three months.

Figure 6.5. A lung scan on a patient with pulmonary embolism reveals perfusion defects in the right lower and left upper lobes. The chest radiograph was normal.

Embolism of Lobar or Segmental Arteries— With Infarction

As already mentioned, pulmonary infarction only occurs after some 15 per cent of embolic episodes. This is to be expected considering the dual blood supply from pulmonary and bronchial vessels. It is more common in patients with a raised left atrial pressure. Of some further importance has been the recognition that not all infarcts seen on the plain chest radiograph represent areas of necrotic tissues; many are so-called 'reversible infarcts', representing areas of haemorrhage without cellular necrosis. The clinical features may be more suggestive of the diagnosis than in the group without infarction. Notwithstanding this, the diagnosis is frequently in doubt. The radiographic features are described below.

There is usually a pulmonary opacity, which is classically situated in the lower lobes and often lies adjacent to one or two pleural surfaces (Figure 6.6). Any fresh peripheral parapleural shadow should be considered as possibly caused by a pulmonary infarct, particularly in debilitated and postoperative patients (Figures 6.7 and 6.8). Elevation of the diaphragm on the affected side may occur before development of this opacity. The triangular shape of the shadow is a myth. It may, however, have a hump-like configuration, convex medially (Figure 6.8). The opacity may develop

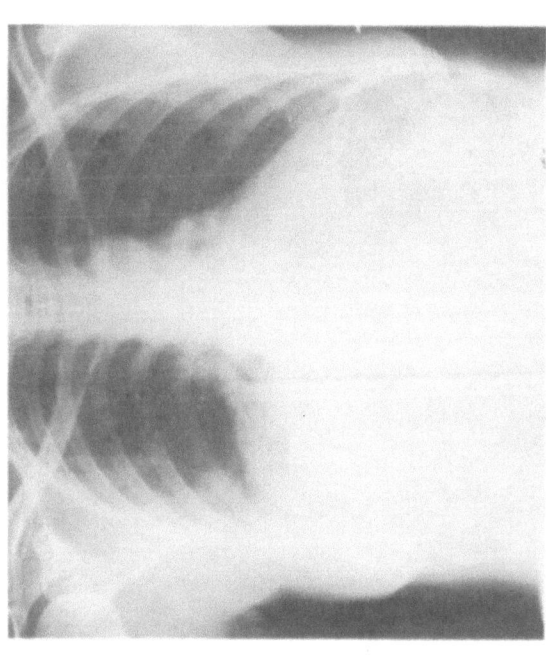

Figure 6.6. Chest radiograph eight days after an abdominal operation. The patient had haemoptysis. A lung scan revealed multiple perfusion defects in both lungs suggesting that the right lower lobe consolidation was caused by pulmonary infarction rather than pneumonia.

61

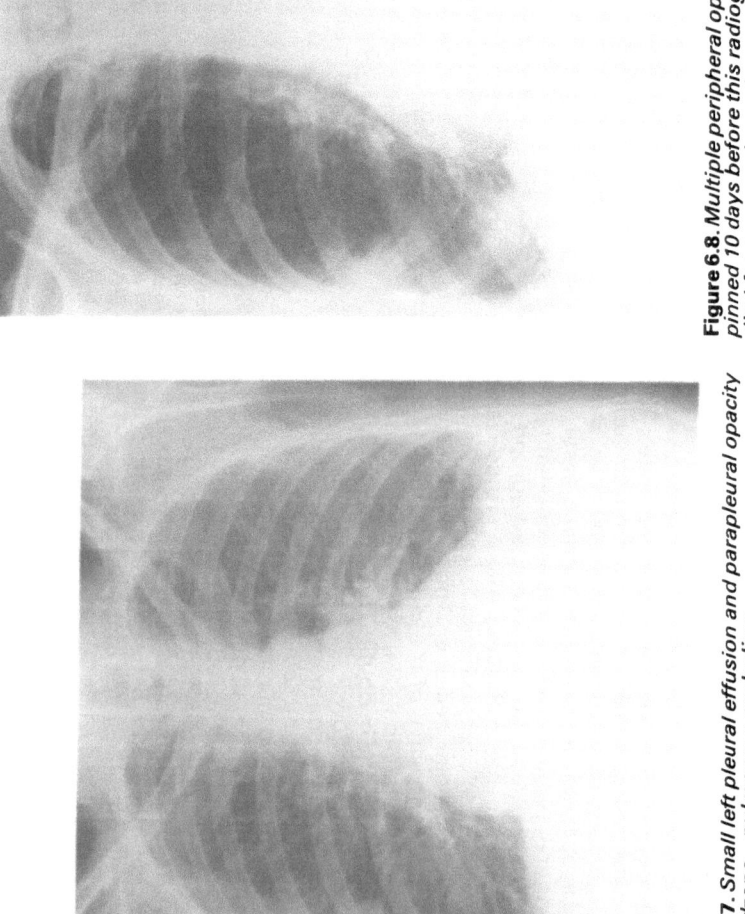

Figure 6.8. Multiple peripheral opacities. The patient had a hip pinned 10 days before this radiograph was taken. The patient died from a massive pulmonary embolism two days later.

Figure 6.7. Small left pleural effusion and parapleural opacity right midzone—pulmonary embolism.

over several days. It usually disappears completely within one to four weeks (the reversible infarct) but may leave a residual horizontal line shadow (Figure 6.9), usually situated just above the diaphragm, abutting against the pleura, and some 3 to 5 cm in length. Very occasionally, multiple pulmonary shadows, which may be surprisingly discrete and resemble metastases, are caused by infarcts.

Small pleural effusions are common. Large effusions, which are often bloody, sometimes occur. Enlargement of the descending pulmonary artery to the involved lobe is an associated finding which may further allow differentiation from a pneumonia. It is important to realise that there are no pathognomonic radiographic signs. Serial films and an awareness of the possibility are important. A perfusion scan will not differentiate between an infarct and any other pulmonary or pleural opacity. However, the demonstration on the scan of other perfusion defects corresponding to the 'normal' areas on the chest radiograph, allows a presumptive diagnosis to be made. If an absolute diagnosis is required, pulmonary angiography may be performed.

Multiple Small Peripheral Emboli

Multiple small emboli are probably quite common and often go unrecognized. Occasionally, when recurrent,

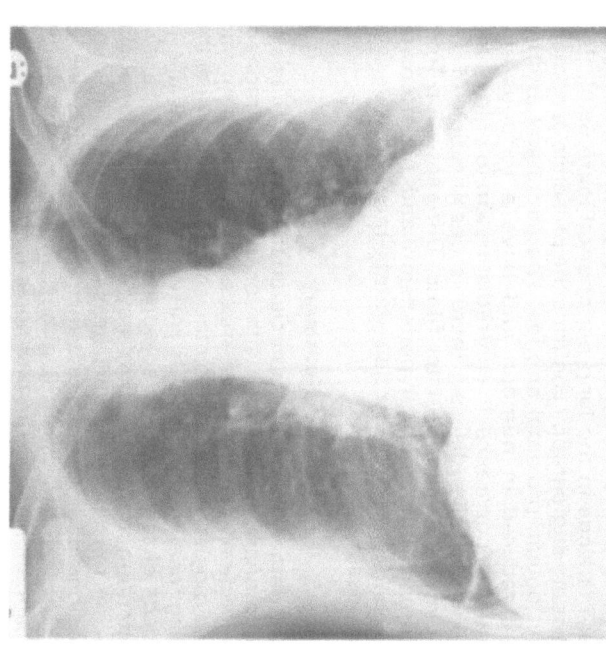

Figure 6.9. *Basal line shadows indicative of healed infarcts.*

63

they may produce the clinical picture of progressive pulmonary arterial hypertension. The chest radiograph reveals cardiomegaly with dilatation of the main pulmonary artery. The hilar and proximal pulmonary arteries are prominent and there are diminished vascular markings in the lung periphery (Figure 6.10). Pulmonary angiography confirms the presence of dilated, but patent, proximal arteries. The peripheral arteries are reduced in number, and have a tortuous and pruned appearance. In contradistinction to pulmonary veno-occlusive disease, there is opacification of the pulmonary veins on later films. Differentiation from primary pulmonary hypertension and hypertension secondary to intracardiac shunts may, however, be impossible.

Summary

In summary, it can be appreciated that the diagnosis of pulmonary embolism, with or without pulmonary infarction, can only be made if the clinician and radiologist responsible for the case constantly bear the diagnosis in mind and if correct and prompt use is made of scanning and angiographic facilities. Careful attention to the plain film may suggest the diagnosis. Scans must be interpreted in association with the chest radiograph and in congnisance of their limitations.

The time to perform either angiography or lung scanning is when the diagnosis is first suspected.

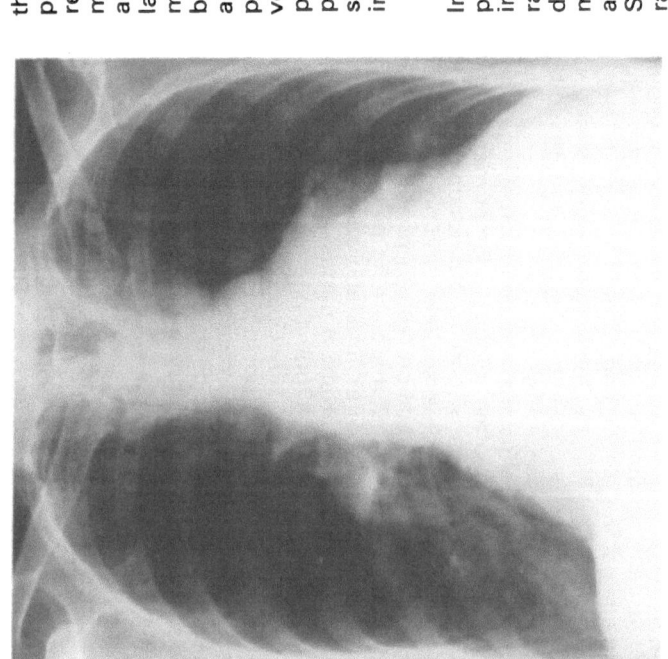

Figure 6.10. *Pulmonary hypertension with enlarged proximal pulmonary arteries.*

7. Diffuse Pulmonary Disease

A considerable diagnostic problem is posed by the chest radiograph with disseminate pulmonary opacities. Sometimes the diagnosis is obvious, e.g. multiple metastases in a patient with known malignancy, or suggested by the prevailing circumstances, e.g. a routine film in a coalface worker.

Frequently, however, a 'spot' diagnosis is impossible but careful appraisal of the radiographic appearances and then correlation with the relevant clinical information may narrow considerably an otherwise wide field of possible diagnoses.

For purposes of discussion, diffuse pulmonary disease may be grouped according to the size and opacity of the densities and their pattern of distribution (Table 7.1).

A variety of terms has been applied to the different radiographic patterns. Generally it is preferable to use simple descriptive terms, recognizing that these do not connote specific pathological processes. Attempts have been made to correlate the radiographic appearances with pathological processes which are primarily alveolar or interstitial in form. Although occasionally possible, many radiologists either find this too difficult a correlation to achieve, or believe it to be so frequently impossible as to be of no practical value.

Disseminate Small Shadows

The most difficult group to deal with is disseminate small shadows. A daunting list of some 83 causes has been given by Scadding.* Perfect quality radiographs are essential. Underpenetrated or expiratory films of *normal* lungs may appear abnormal and diffuse pulmonary disease may be simulated.

Miliary Pattern

The miliary pattern is composed of disseminate tiny discrete opacities which are mostly 2 to 3 mm in size.

Table 7.1. Diffuse pulmonary disease.

Disseminate small shadows
  Miliary pattern
  Disseminate high radio-opacity nodules
  Reticulonodular shadowing
Disseminate large shadows

* Scadding (1952), *Tubercle*, **33**, 352.

They are usually not associated with any accompanying line shadows and there is no tendency to coalesce. There is a fairly even distribution of lesions throughout both lungs. This pattern is classically observed in miliary tuberculosis, when the patient is usually ill (Figure 7.1). It is also the typical appearance of early silicosis (Figure 7.2) and other rarer inorganic pneumoconioses, such as berylliosis and siderosis. Unlike miliary tuberculosis, the patient is usually well.

Miliary shadowing is an unusual manifestation of sarcoidosis. Although rare, it is a recognized appearance in metastatic tumour spread, and is said to be more common with papillary thyroid carcinoma and chorion carcinoma. It is the classic appearance of primary haemosiderosis and is also seen in pulmonary haemosiderosis secondary to mitral valve disease. The cardiac configuration in the latter makes the diagnosis obvious. In patients from North America, such fungal infections as histoplasmosis, coccidioidomycosis and cryptococcosis should always be remembered, as should schistosomiasis in patients who have been resident abroad.

Disseminate High Radio-opacity Nodules

The appearance of disseminate high radio-opacity nodules occurs in only a few disorders, some of which are exceedingly rare. However, a working acquaint-

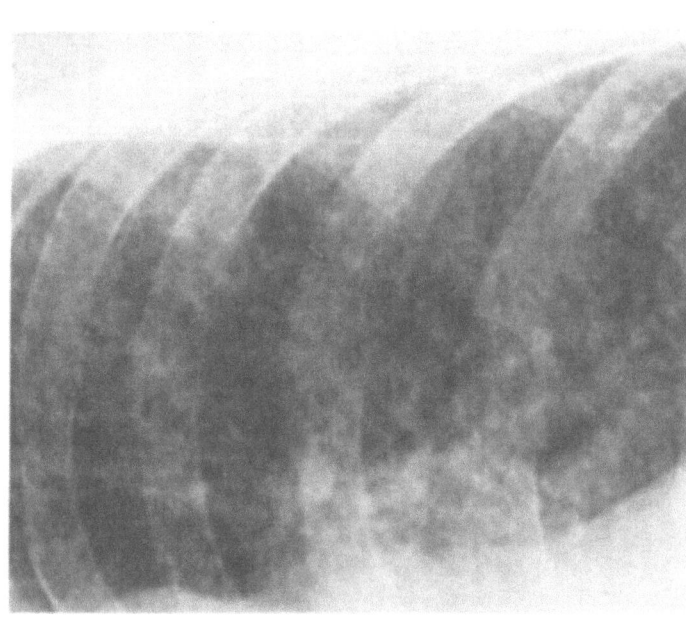

Figure 7.1. *Miliary tuberculosis.*

ance with these is useful because a specific diagnosis can often be made. Scattered, small nodular calcifications, (2 to 3 mm in diameter) are seen in healed tuberculosis (Figure 7.3) and some years after chickenpox pneumonia (Figure 7.4). They are usually more evenly distributed throughout the lungs in the latter. An identical appearance is seen as a late manifestation of histoplasmosis (a much commoner disease than either tuberculosis or chickenpox pneumonia in parts of North America).

Small nodular shadows of bony density in the lower lobes are seen in the metaplastic pulmonary ossification associated with long-standing mitral valve disease.

Of a lower radio-opacity are the finer pinpoint shadows of haemosiderosis. Equally tiny densities, but of a much higher radio-opacity, are characteristic of alveolar microlithiasis. The chest radiograph is diagnostic.

Certain occupational disorders caused by the inhalation of particulate matter of high atomic number do not provoke a fibrotic reaction and cause no pulmonary disability, unlike silica and asbestos fibres. Such disorders include stannosis (tin smelting), baritosis (barium inhalation), talcosis (talc inhalation) and siderosis (iron welding).

Fine miliary mottling is sometimes seen on films taken following a lymphogram.

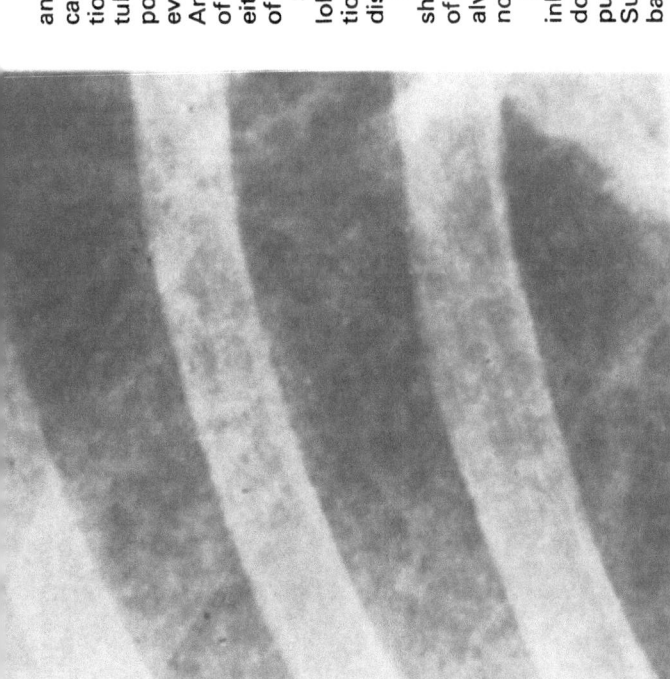

Figure 7.2. Silicosis. In the more common pneumoconiosis the opacities are often not as well defined. This patient was a sandblaster.

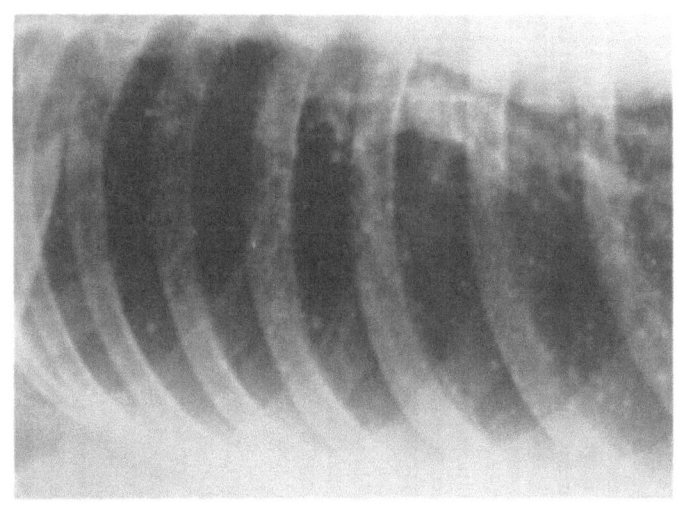

Figure 7.4. *Small evenly distributed calcific nodules. Residue of chicken pox pneumonia.*

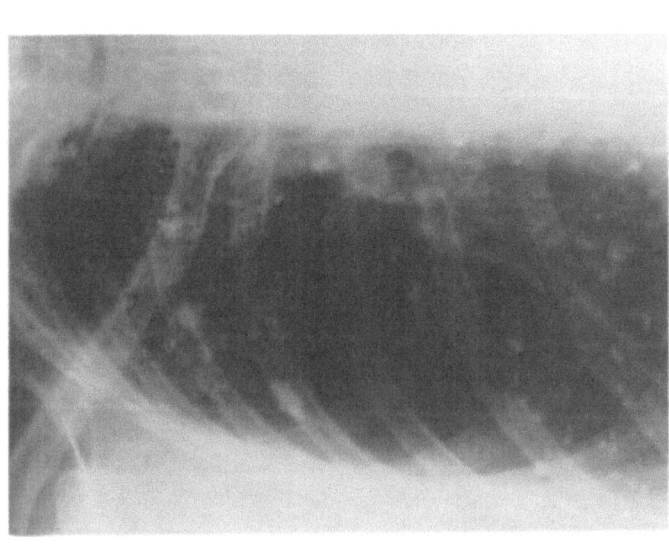

Figure 7.3. *Scattered calcifications of uneven size and distribution. Tuberculosis.*

Reticulonodular Shadowing

Reticulonodular shadowing implies the presence of nodular shadows, which may be well or ill defined, in association with a linear or reticular pattern. Either the nodular or linear component may predominate. Early on there may be simply an increased prominence of the normal lung markings. Later a honeycomb pattern may be observed. This is a descriptive term of an appearance which may be caused by superimposition and summation of tiny nodular shadows. It does not necessarily imply the presence of a 'honeycomb lung', as defined by the pathologist. The more important causes of reticulonodular shadowing are listed in Table 7.2.

Although a diagnosis is not possible from a single film, the field can be narrowed by attention to radiographic features and to clinical data.

Table 7.2. Causes of diffuse reticulonodular shadowing.

Sarcoidosis
Inorganic pneumoconioses
 Silicosis
 Coal worker's pneumoconiosis
 Asbestosis
Cryptogenic fibrosing alveolitis
Scleroderma
Asbestosis
Rheumatoid disease
Acute extrinsic allergic alveolitis
 Farmer's lung
 Mushroom worker's lung
 Bird fancier's lung
Neoplasms
 Haematogenous metastases
 Alveolar cell carcinoma
 Lymphomas
 Lymphangitis carcinomatosa
Eosinophilic lung states
Bronchopulmonary aspergillosis
Polyarteritis nodosa
Drugs
Pulmonary oedema
Intrapulmonary haemorrhage (Goodpasture's)
Tuberose sclerosis
Histiocytosis X
Neurofibromatosis
Lymphangiomyomatosis
Alveolar proteinosis
Infections
 Tuberculosis
 Viral and mycoplasma pneumonias
 Fungal infections
 Opportunistic infections
Chronic aspiration pneumonias (including lipoid pneumonias)
Cystic fibrosis
Widespread bronchiectasis

Differentiating Radiographic Features

Distribution. A predominantly lower lobe distribution is in keeping with asbetosis, aspiration pneumonia,

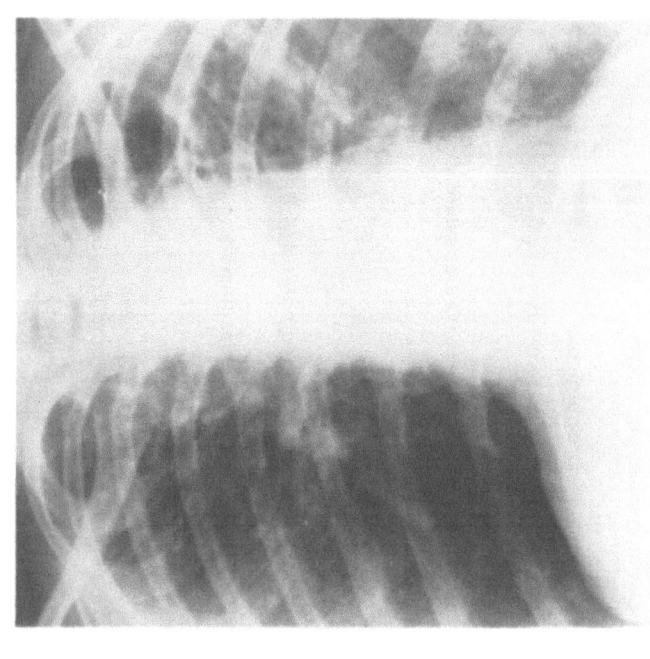

Figure 7.6. Ill defined upper lobe shadowing with shrinkage. There is also a cavity at the left apex. Tuberculosis.

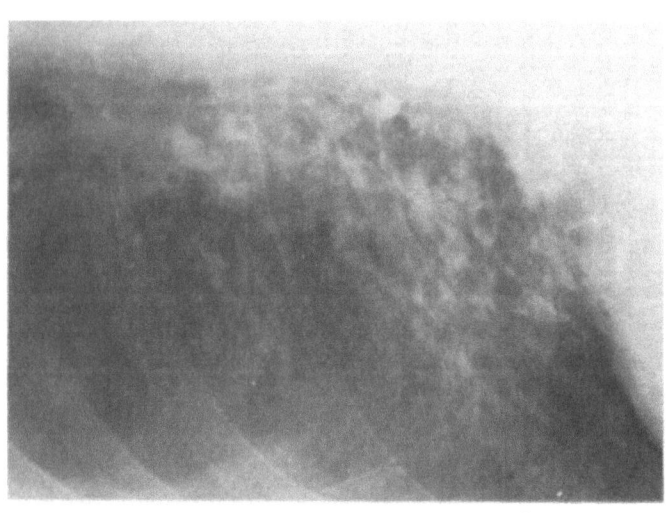

Figure 7.5. Ill defined predominantly basal shadowing. Bronchiectasis.

bronchiectasis (Figure 7.5), cryptogenic fibrosing alveolitis and scleroderma. Ill defined nodular shadows in association with upper lobe cavitation should suggest the possibility of tuberculosis (Figure 7.6). Upper lobe shrinkage also occurs as a late manifestation in bird-fancier's lung, sarcoidosis (Figure 7.7), bronchopulmonary aspergillosis, with advanced coalworker's pneumoconiosis and in ankylosing spondylitis.

Pulmonary oedema, alveolar proteinosis and Pneumocystis carinii pneumonia often begin as perihilar shadowing (Figure 7.8).

Pleural effusions occur with many of the disorders listed, but most notably may be seen with pulmonary oedema, lymphangitis carcinomatosa, lymphomas, rheumatoid lung, and lupus erythematosus. Pleural plaques are a feature of asbestosis, although they are not a necessary accompaniment. A pleural reaction is notably uncommon in cryptogenic fibrosing alveolitis, sarcoidosis, scleroderma and histiocytosis X. The last named is not infrequently associated with a spontaneous pneumothorax, which is also a late feature of Pneumocystis carinii pneumonia (Figure 7.9).

Lung volume is invariably increased in cystic fibrosis (Figure 7.10), in contrast to fibrosing alveolitis, where a reduction in lung volume often occurs.

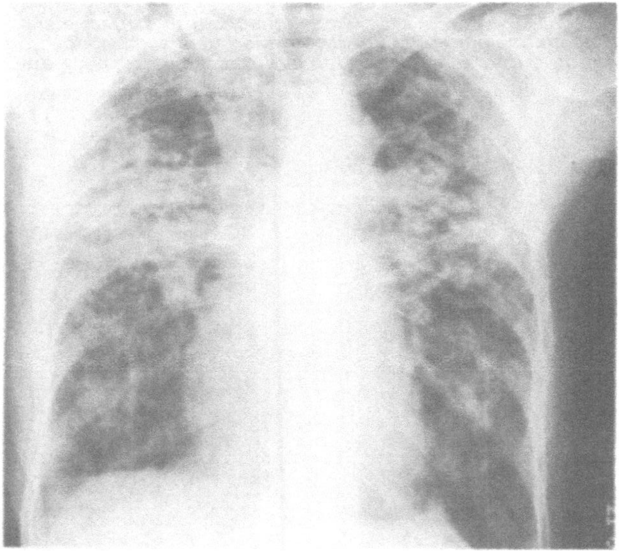

Figure 7.7 Sarcoidosis with pulmonary fibrosis, most pronounced in the mid and upper zones.

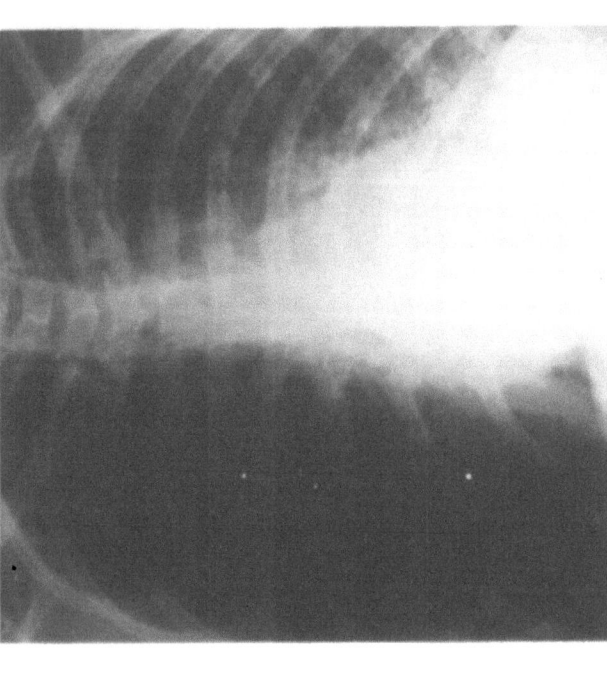

Figure 7.9. *Histiocytosis. Reticular shadowing with a honey–comb appearance. Left pneumothorax with mediastinal shift. This is a feature of histiocytosis.*

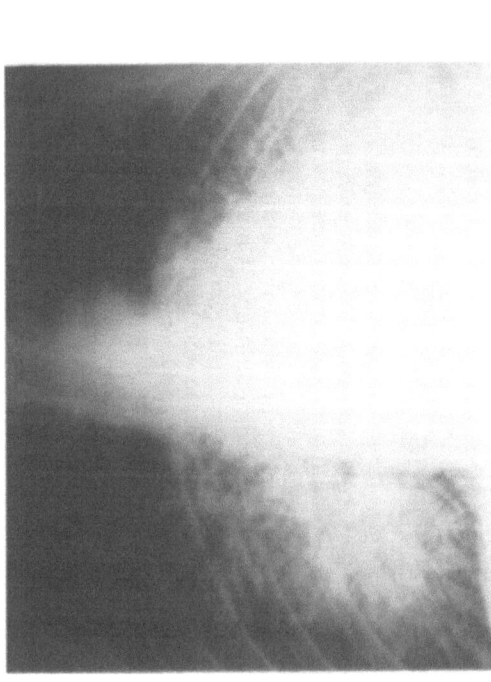

Figure 7.8. *Batswing pattern of pulmonary oedema. Note the enlarged heart.*

Hilar adenopathy occurs in many cases of sarcoidosis (Figure 7.11). Berylliosis is indistinguishable. In silicosis and the lymphomas the hilar component may also be prominent. Tuberculosis and fungal infections occasionally cause impressive and frequently asymmetrical, mediastinal adenopathy (Figure 7.12).

Septal lines are commonly present in lymphangitis carcinomatosa (Figure 7.13). They are also frequently seen in pulmonary oedema (Figure 7.14) and silicosis and are not uncommon in fibrosing alveolitis and sarcoidosis.

Ring shadows are seen in bronchiectasis (Figures 7.5 and 7.15), histiocytosis X and tuberose sclerosis when they may amount to bullae.

A honeycomb appearance is frequently seen in these diseases and also in cryptogenic fibrosing alveolitis (Figure 7.16), scleroderma, asbestosis and rheumatoid lung.

Abnormalities in the cardiovascular structures should be noted – cardiomegaly is the usual accompaniment of pulmonary oedema, secondary to left heart failure. There is usually diversion of blood to the upper lobes. Pericardial effusion is a feature of systemic lupus erythematosus.

A predominantly nodular pattern is seen in silicosis,

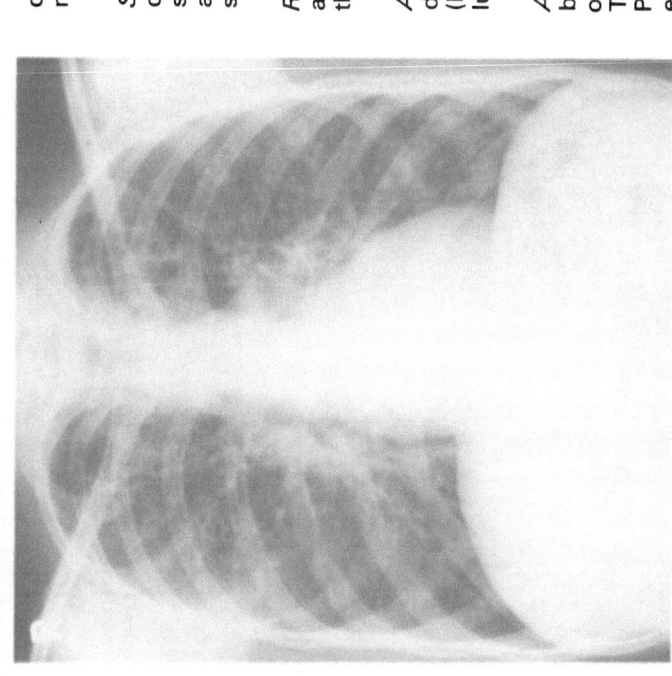

Figure 7.10. Cystic fibrosis. Coarse linear markings and ill defined nodules. Prominent hilar shadows.

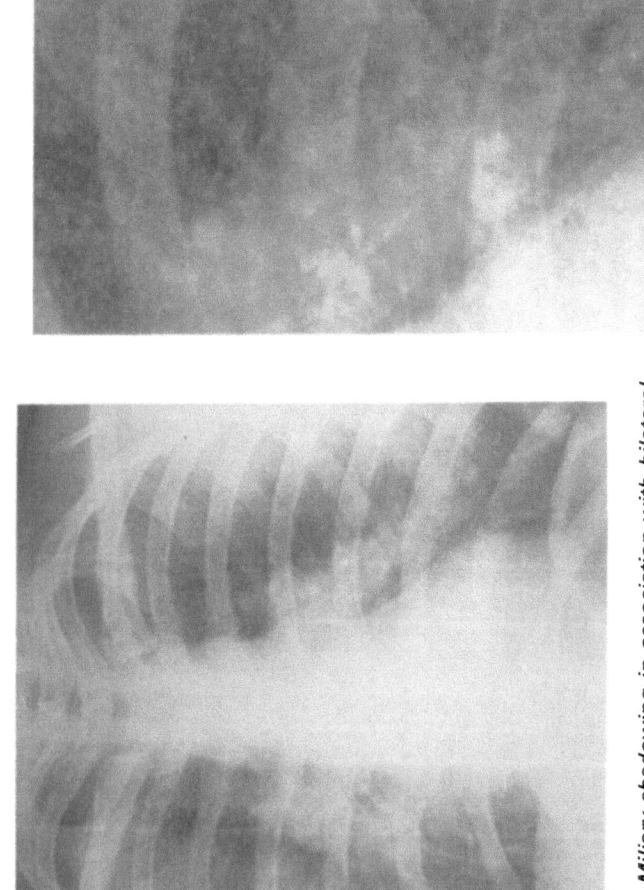

Figure 7.11. Miliary shadowing in association with bilateral hilar adenopathy. Sarcoidosis.

Figure 7.12. Ill defined nodular shadowing with left hilar adenopathy. Tuberculous bronchopneumonia.

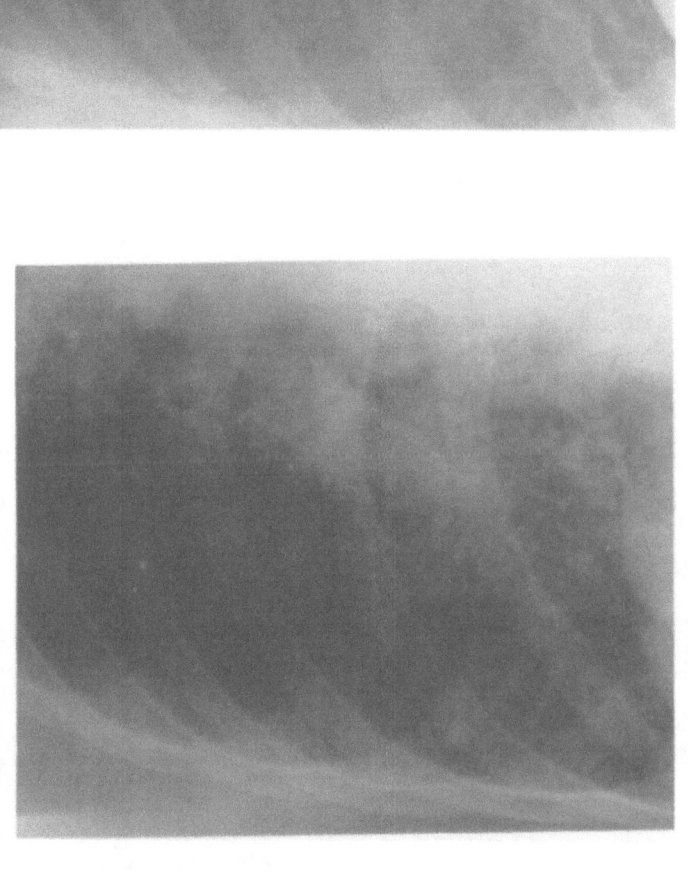

Figure 7.13. *Lymphangitis carcinomatosa showing abundant septal lines and a small pleural effusion.*

Figure 7.14. *Pulmonary oedema. The main abnormality is an abundance of septal lines.*

75

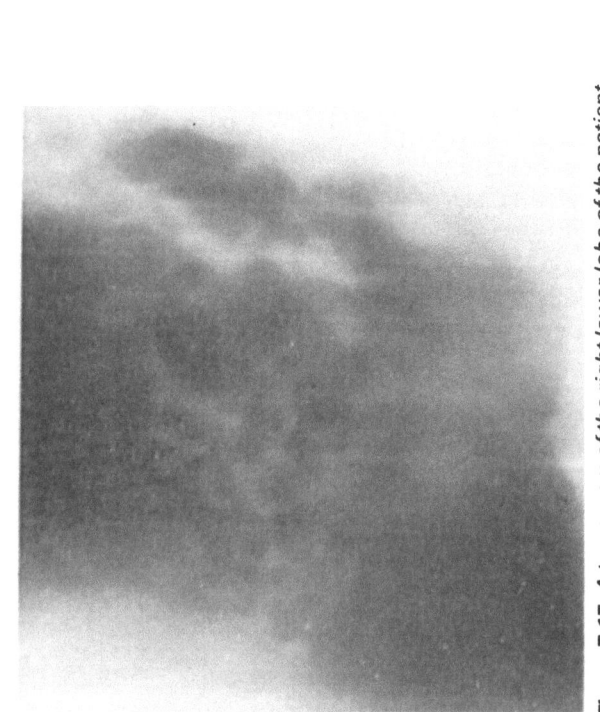

Figure 7.15. A tomogram of the right lower lobe of the patient in Figure 7.5 reveals multiple ring shadows typical of bronchiectasis.

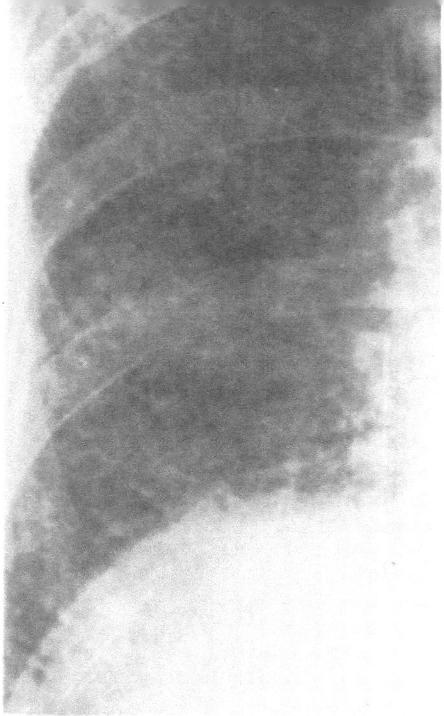

Figure 7.16. Reticular shadowing giving a honeycomb appearance in a patient with cryptogenic fibrosing alveolitis.

sarcoidosis (Figure 7.17) and with haematogenous metastases (alveolar cell carcinoma). The nodules are usually fairly well defined and vary in size from 3 to 5 mm. Larger nodules may be seen with metastases. As silicosis and sarcoidosis progress, there is usually an increasing linear component. Diffuse pulmonary fibrosis, whatever its cause, is characterized by a predominantly reticular appearance, which starts as a barely recognizable blurring of the normal lung markings. Serial films will establish whether or not there has been any progression of the disease over weeks or months, and may also help in suggesting the nature of the disease by the pattern of change.

Finally, some attention should be paid to the bones of the thorax. Characteristic lesions may be seen in histiocytosis X and destructive areas provide the clue to the diagnosis in disseminated malignancy.

Differentiating Clinical Features

It is not desirable to report on chest radiographs of this sort in a clinical vacuum. Marked abnormalities on the film are sometimes seen in symptomless patients—sarcoidosis or a pneumoconiosis are by far the most likely causes. An occupational history is obviously of paramount importance (Figure 7.18). The necessary information may only be obtained with close questioning and through a thorough knowledge of

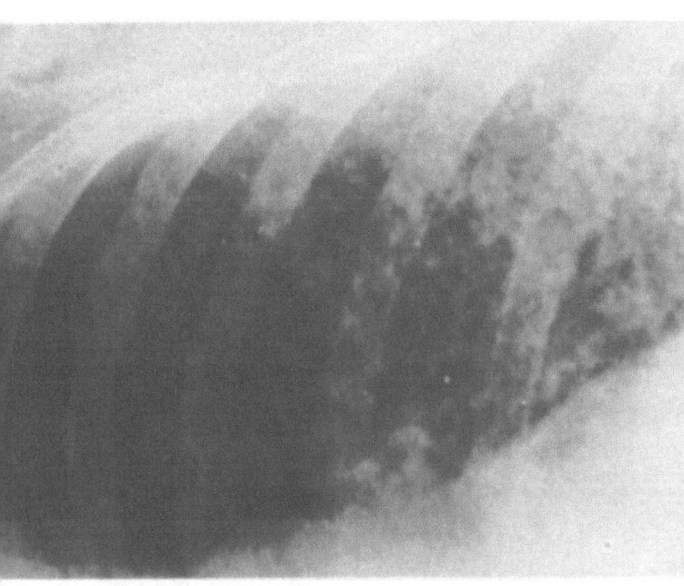

Figure 7.17. Widespread nodules 3 to 5 mm in size. Metastatic pancreatic carcinoma.

local factors. Although most patients with pulmonary infections are ill and febrile, those with an altered immunity may exhibit quite florid pulmonary changes with a minimum of symptoms (Figure 7.19).

Drug-induced disease is increasingly common and readily overlooked; busulphan, nitrofurantoin (Figure 7.20), the sulphonamides and hexamethonium are drugs which affect the lung, but there are many others in addition. Inhalation of noxious gases or fumes should be considered in the acutely ill patient with diffuse pulmonary shadowing. Finger-clubbing and basal crepitations are commonly observed in cryptogenic fibrosing alveolitis. They are not a feature of tuberose sclerosis or histiocytosis, which also produce a honeycomb appearance in the lung. Dyspnoea is a feature of diffuse pulmonary fibrosis and is an invariable accompaniment of lymphangitis carcinomatosa, while wheeze may be present in eosinophilic lung states, such as bronchopulmonary aspergillosis and polyarteritis nodosa. Dysphagia suggests the likelihood of scleroderma or aspiration pneumonia (Figures 7.21 and 7.22). A history of arthralgia obtained in a patient with fibrosing alveolitis suggests rheumatoid arthritis. Arthralgia also occurs in polyarteritis nodosa, lupus erythematosus and sarcoidosis.

Sputum examination is sometimes helpful. Blood and skin tests should be performed as indicated.

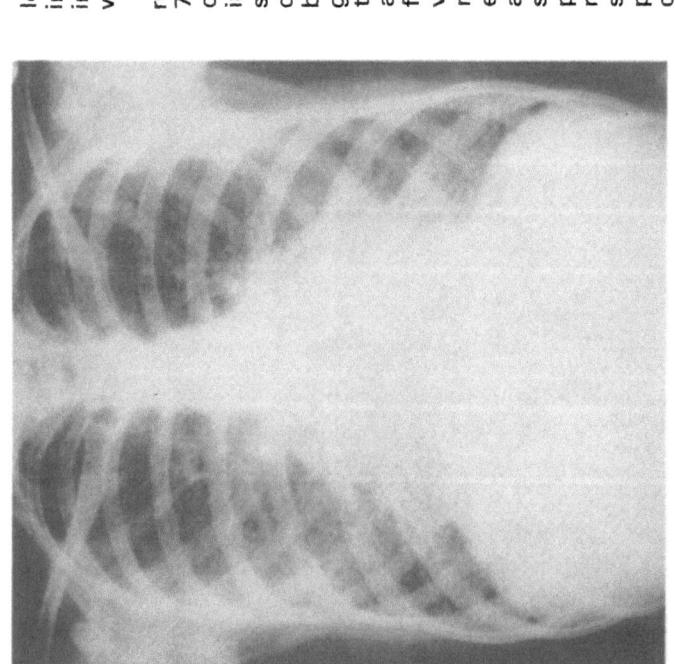

Figure 7.18. *Acute extrinsic allergic alveolitis in a mushroom picker.*

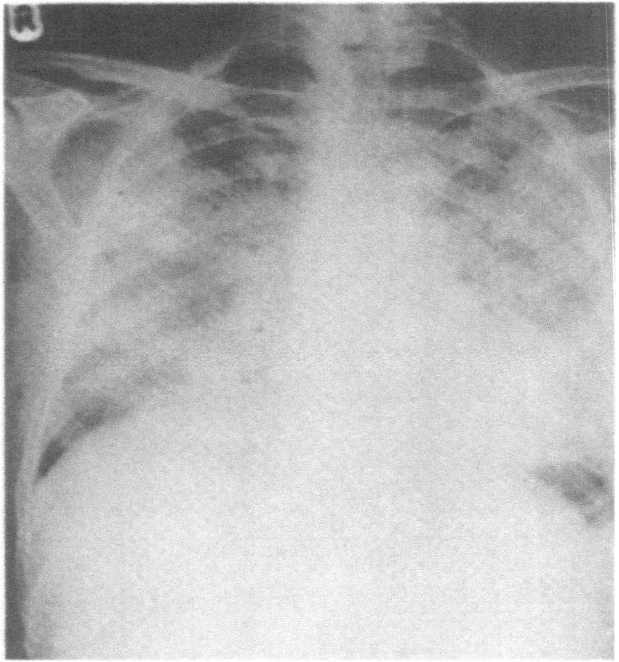

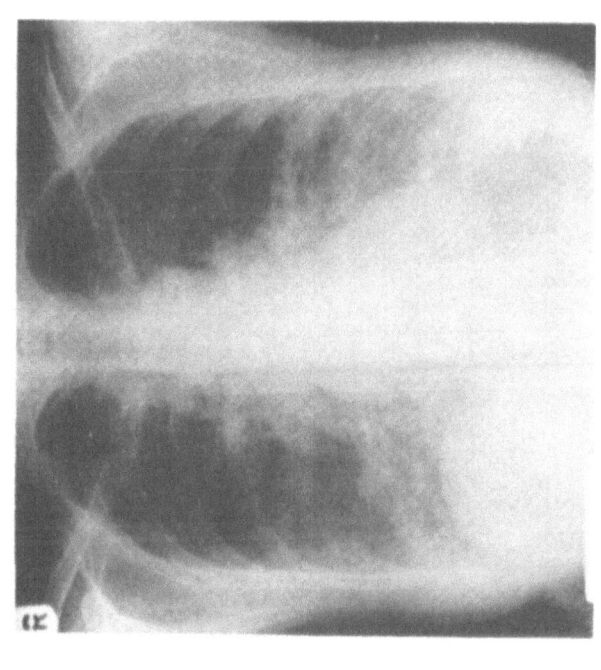

Figure 7.19. Pneumocystis pneumonia in a patient with leukaemia.

Figure 7.20. Ill defined diffuse pulmonary shadowing caused by nitrofurantoin hypersensitivity.

79

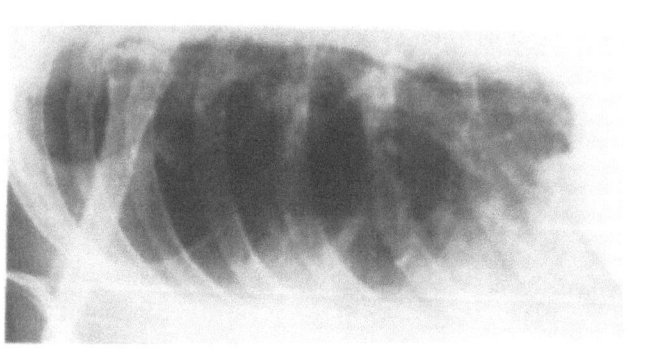

Figure 7.21. Chronic aspiration pneumonia.

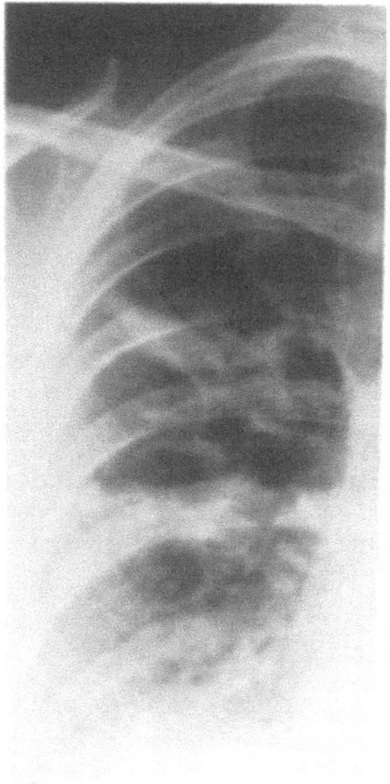

Figure 7.22. Eosinophilic infiltration in an asthmatic patient.

Biopsy of lymph nodes, liver or lung may be required.

Disseminate Large Shadows

Disseminated large shadows comprise multiple disseminate opacities which are more than 1 cm in diameter. The causes of such an appearance are listed in Table 7.3.

Table 7.3. Disseminate large shadows.

Metastases
Pulmonary infarcts
Pyaemic abscesses
Hydatid cysts
Rheumatoid nodules
Wegener's granuloma
Eosinophilic lung states
Multiple arteriovenous malformations

Haematogenous metastases account for most cases (Figure 7.23). The opacities are usually, but not invariably, well defined. Squamous carcinoma metastases occasionally cavitate. Calcification within the lesions is not seen, although metastases from an osteogenic sarcoma may ossify. Disseminate shadows are an uncommon feature of the lymphomas. Hydatid cysts are usually well defined. They do not calcify and may mimic metastases very closely.
Multiple pulmonary infarcts are usually ill defined

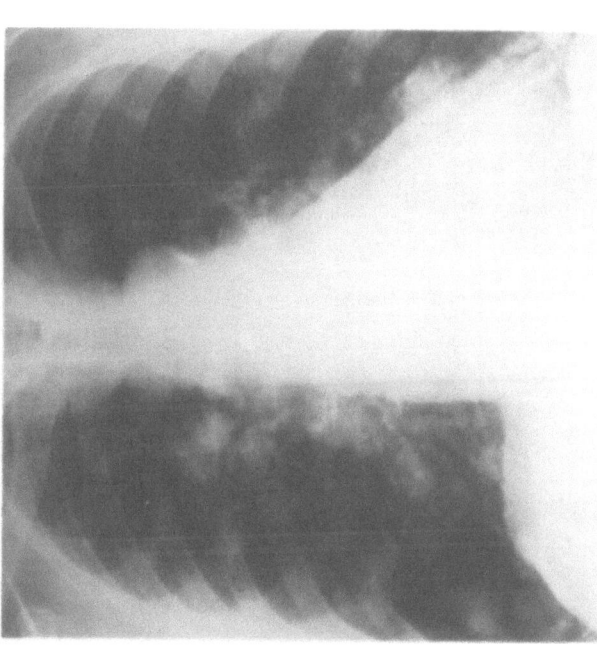

Figure 7.23. *Typical appearance of widespread pulmonary metastases.*

81

and few in number (Figure 7.24). The history is often suggestive. A very similar radiographic appearance is also seen with multiple pyaemic abscesses and is sometimes observed in eosinophilic lung states, particularly in asthmatics. Awareness of the condition, the history and a blood eosinophilia allow a fairly ready diagnosis.

Wegener's granuloma and rheumatoid arthritis cause disseminate, irregular or ill defined opacities, which occasionally cavitate. Multiple arteriovenous malformations and fungal infections are very rare causes of this pattern.

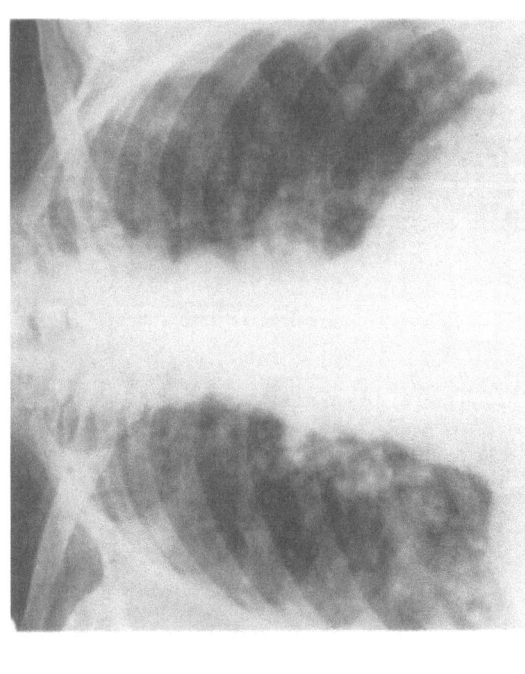

Figure 7.24. Multiple pulmonary infarcts mimicking haematogenous metastases.

8. Pleural Lesions

Pleural lesions are common. They occasionally cause confusion if the observer is not aware of their ability to produce unusual appearances. However, use of basic radiological principles will usually lead to the correct diagnosis.

Pleural Effusions

Large pleural effusions are usually obvious on clinical grounds. The chest radiograph confirms the diagnosis, and often determines whether there is any underlying pulmonary abnormality. Occasionally, it may be possible to suggest a pathological diagnosis. Although the natural elasticity of the lung causes the lung on the affected side to recoil towards its hilum, there is usually some shift of the mediastinal structures away from the side of an effusion (Figure 8.1). If the mediastinal structures remain central despite a large effusion, underlying pulmonary collapse, frequently caused by bronchial obstruction, should be considered. This is a common presentation of bronchial carcinomas. Over-

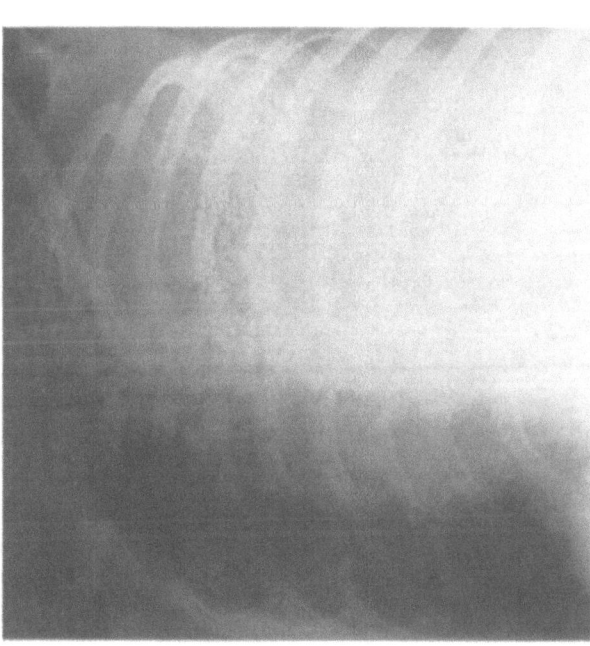

Figure 8.1. *Massive left pleural effusion with shift of the mediastinal structures to the right.*

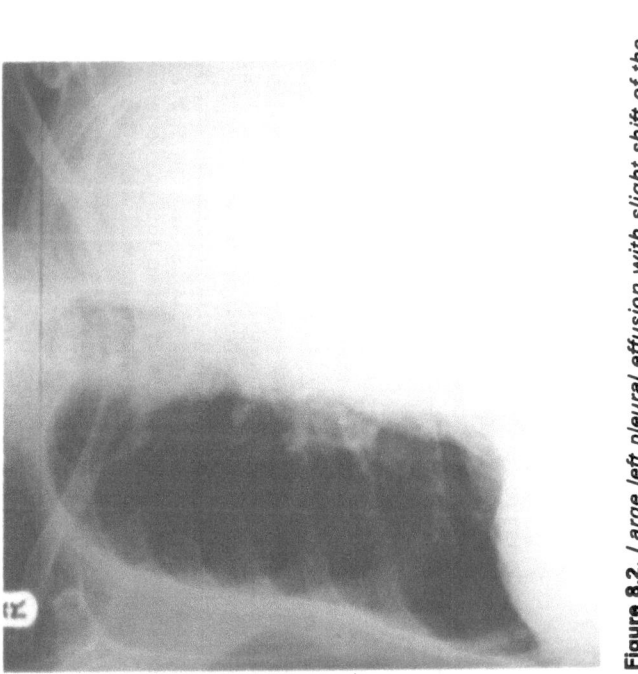

Figure 8.2. Large left pleural effusion with slight shift of the mediastinal structures to the left implying underlying pulmonary collapse. Tomography revealed complete occlusion of the left main bronchus. The ultimate diagnosis was bronchial carcinoma.

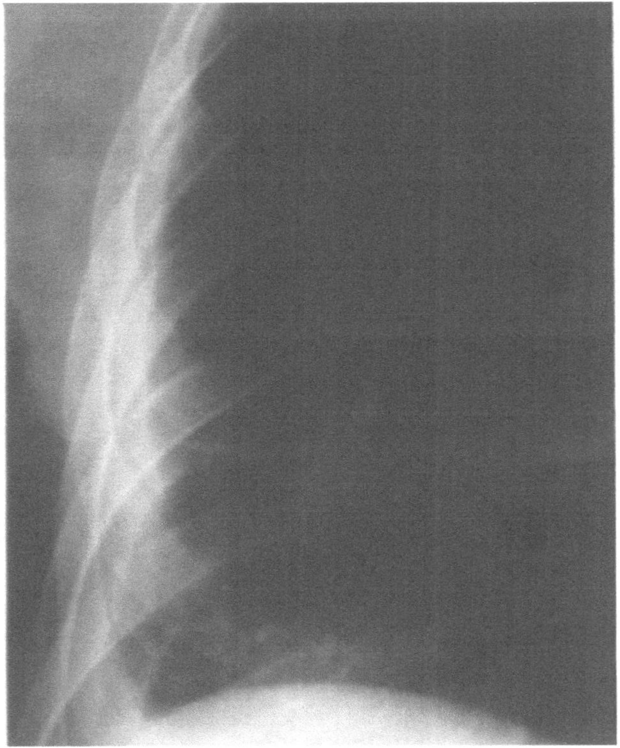

Figure 8.3. Small pleural effusion demonstrated by decubitus film (viewed in the upright position).

penetrated films or tomograms will usually show the obstructed bronchus (Figure 8.2). Conversely, an air bronchogram on these films excludes an underlying bronchial obstruction.

It is sometimes impossible to draw any conclusions about pathological involvement of the underlying lung, because one cannot 'see through' the effusion. However, if well-penetrated supine views are obtained, fluid will usually pass towards the apex of the lung, allowing the lower lobe to be seen more clearly. Any pathological process therein may be more readily detected. Small quantities of pleural fluid are frequently not seen on the PA film. Effusions collect first beneath the lung and in the costophrenic and costo-vertebral recesses. Blunting of the costovertebral angle on the lateral film may therefore be the only evidence of a small effusion. Very small effusions (50 to 100 ml) may be detected by decubitus views (Figure 8.3). The first evidence of an effusion on the PA film is obliteration of the costophrenic angles (Figure 8.4). An identical appearance is produced by pleural thickening, and it must be remembered that on a single film it is often impossible to differentiate between a solid, fluid or semifluid pleural reaction.

Simple effusions usually produce a shadow with a concave upper border, shaped as a meniscus. Such an appearance will obviously be present only on films taken in the erect position. Before attempting aspira-

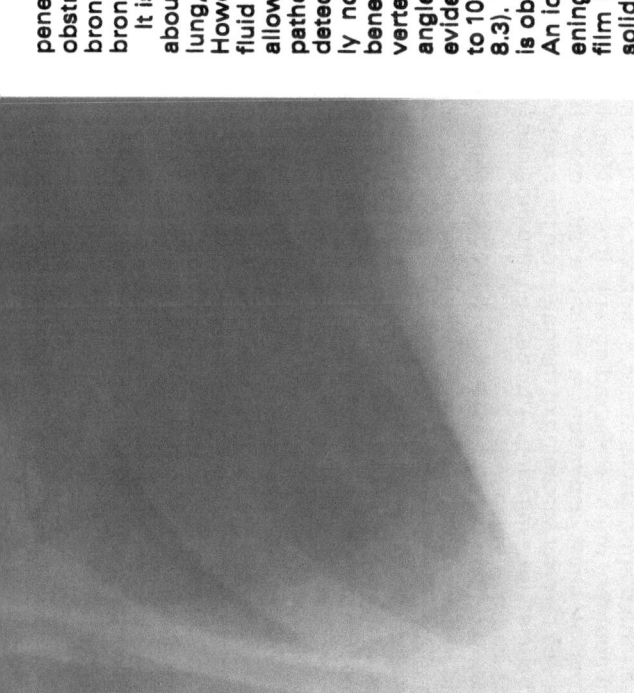

Figure 8.4. *Small pleural effusion obliterating the costophrenic angle, which must always be included in the radiograph.*

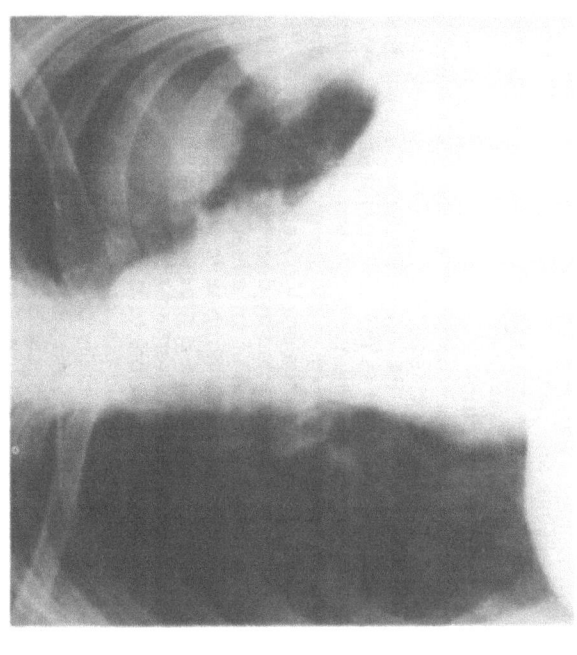

Figure 8.5. *Encysted fluid mimicking pulmonary masses. The patient was in left heart failure.*

tion of any effusion, its position must be accurately determined on PA and lateral views. Erect films are usually taken with the patient standing. Chest aspiration is frequently performed with the patient sitting, when the diaphragm assumes a higher position than that apparent on the chest radiograph. If any difficulty arises at chest aspiration, a suitable site may be marked by prior screening of the patient in the position to be used for aspiration. Alternatively the fluid can be localized by ultrasound.

A not unusual cause of difficulty is the collection of fluid in a subpulmonary position. This is more readily diagnosed on the left, where there is separation of air-containing lung from the gas-filled gastric fundus. The diagnosis is more difficult on the right. The appearance mimics a high hemidiaphragm, but the correct diagnosis is sometimes suggested by the slightly different configuration assumed by this form of effusion. The highest point of its shadow often lies laterally, unlike the diaphragmatic shadow, the highest point of which lies centrally (see Figure 1.11). The diagnosis is confirmed by taking films in the supine or decubitus positions. Rarely the fluid is encysted, in which case such views are of no assistance.

Encysted pleural effusions occur most commonly within the fissures, presenting as the so-called interlobar effusion. In the PA projection they often appear as an ill-defined mass — the pseudotumour appearance (Figures 8.5 and 8.6). With the radiograph beam tangential to the lesion, the effusion assumes its characteristic lenticular shape. Such interlobar effusions are most frequently seen in patients with left heart failure. They may occur in the same place with recurrent episodes of pulmonary oedema.

Encysted effusions may also, though very rarely, collect in a paramediastinal position. They then produce a bizarre cardiac configuration. More commonly, they collect along the lateral aspect of the thorax. They may encase part of the lung and often appear less dense than a pulmonary lesion when viewed en face. It is therefore important to obtain films which allow one to view the lesion tangentially. Lateral and oblique films may be helpful in this respect. When viewed in this way, the medial aspect of the opacity is always well defined, and usually the opacity assumes an elliptical configuration. An empyema (Figure 8.7) or solid pleural mass will produce the same appearance. A fluid level is occasionally seen with the former. However, it more usually denotes attempted aspiration of an effusion or a bronchopleural fistula.

A pleural effusion may be the presenting feature of a subphrenic abscess (see Chapter 10).

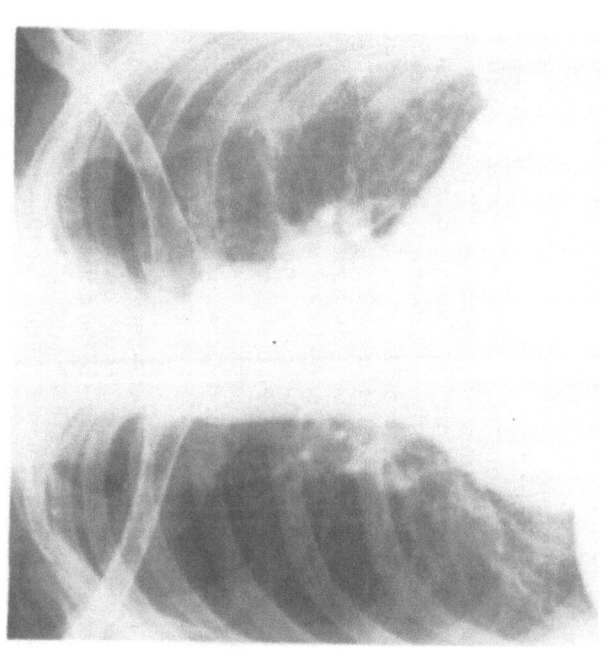

Figure 8.6. *The same patient as in Figure 8.5 after treatment of his heart failure.*

Pleural Neoplasms

Pleural neoplasms may arise from either the parietal or the visceral pleural surfaces. They may present over the convexity of the lung or may arise within an interlobar fissure. The latter, which are rare, are often indistinguishable from an encysted effusion. Mesotheliomas, pleural metastases and pleural fibromas are the most common lesions. Pleural fibromas are usually solitary; they form an obtuse angle with the chest wall when viewed in profile. Fluoroscopy is useful in obtaining correctly positioned films. Pleural metastases and mesotheliomas frequently produce large, bloody pleural effusions. When there is no such accompaniment, however, the appearance is often that of a thickened pleura, sometimes with a rippled medial margin (Figure 8.8). A chronic empyema may give an identical appearance. Pleural tumours may simulate a pleural effusion, from which they can be differentiated by means of ultrasound. Occasionally, metastases and mesotheliomas present as multiple discrete pleural deposits (Figure 8.9).

Tumours arising in or adjacent to the ribs often produce a prominent extrapulmonary soft tissue component. Careful scrutiny of the adjacent ribs is therefore important (Figures 8.10 and 8.11). Metastases and deposits of myeloma (Figure 8.12) are the most common of such lesions, which are rarely mimicked

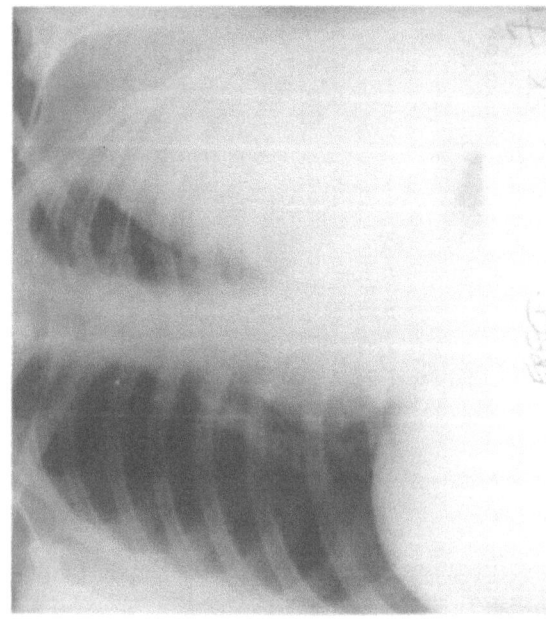

Figure 8.7. *Large empyema with typical elliptical configuration.*

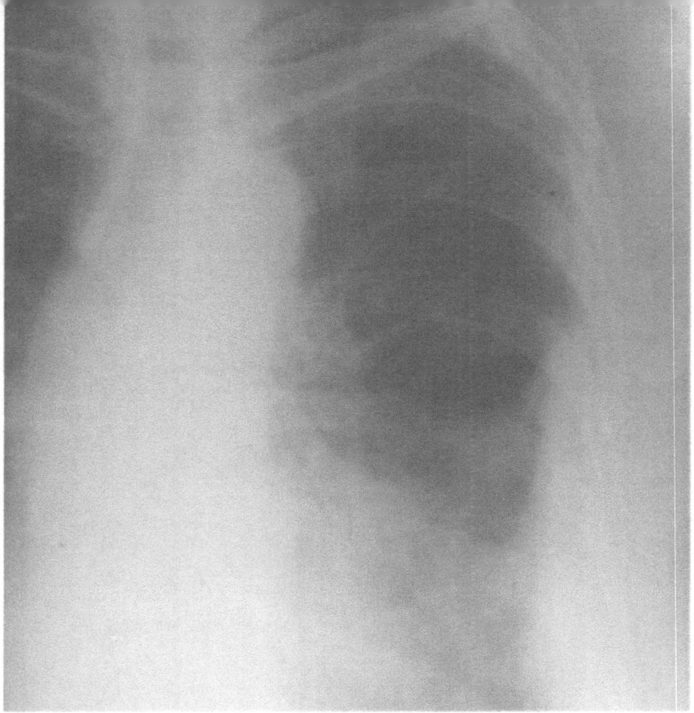

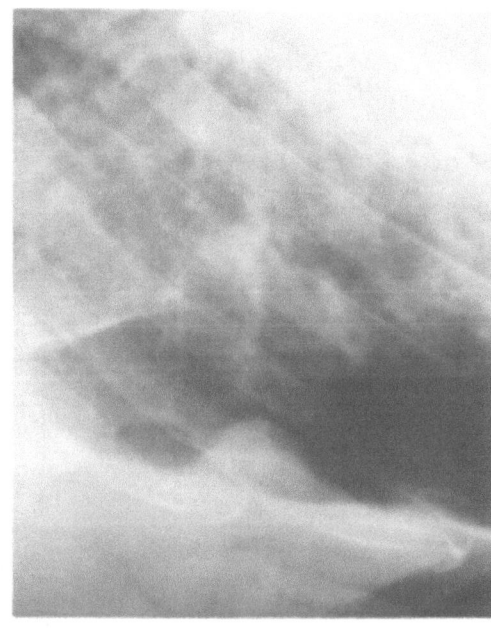

Figure 8.9. *Spot film of a pleural metastasis from a carcinoma of the pancreas. Both lungs were covered by such lesions.*

by fungal diseases. Simple healing rib fractures should not be forgotten as a cause of small extrapulmonary masses, which may be particularly florid in patients taking large doses of steroids or with Cushing's syndrome.

Figure 8.8. *Mesothelioma producing a thickened pleura.*

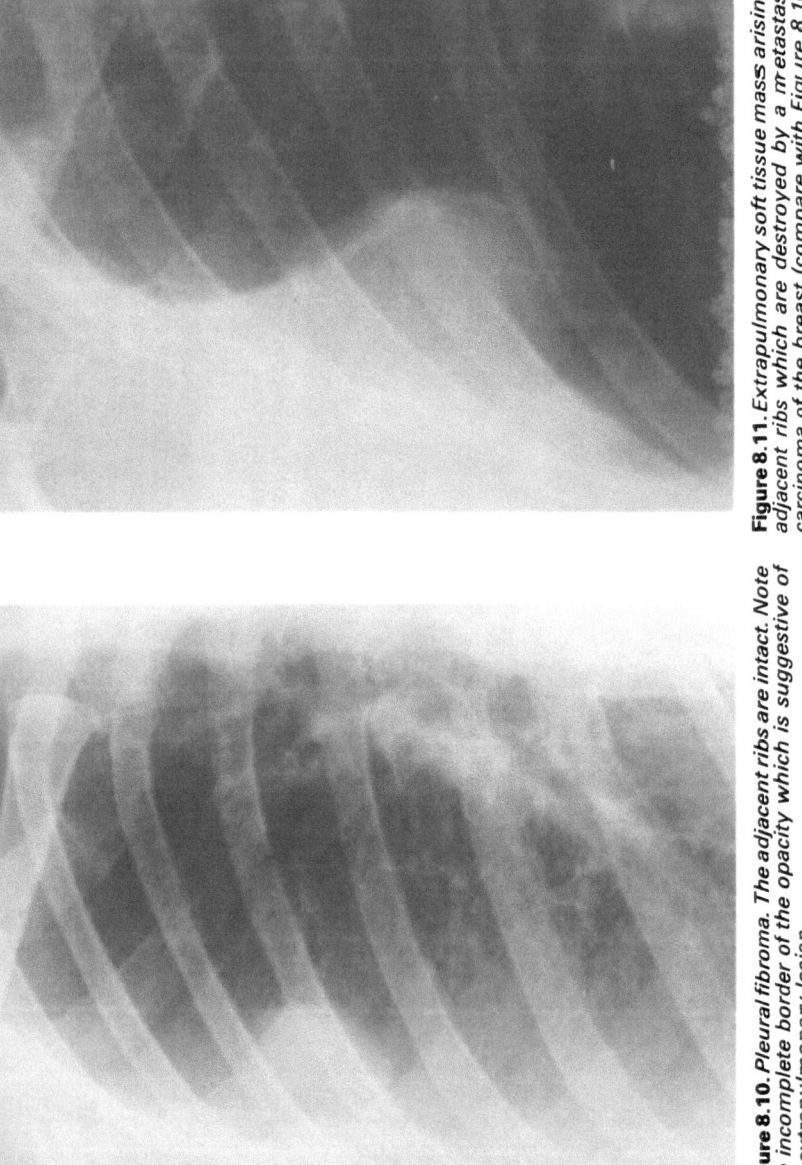

Figure 8.10. Pleural fibroma. The adjacent ribs are intact. Note the incomplete border of the opacity which is suggestive of an extrapulmonary lesion.

Figure 8.11. Extrapulmonary soft tissue mass arising from the adjacent ribs which are destroyed by a metastasis from a carcinoma of the breast (compare with Figure 8.10).

Bilateral apical pleural thickening is common, especially in elderly patients. When a pronounced unilateral apical cap is seen, the possibility of a Pancoast tumour should be considered. Coned films of the posterior aspects of the upper ribs allow careful appraisal of these structures for bony destruction which will confirm the diagnosis (Figure 8.13).

Pneumothorax

The introduction of air into the pleural space, as with fluid, causes the lungs to recoil towards the hilum. The pneumothorax is therefore recognized as a relatively transradiant area bounded medially by the pencilled line of visceral pleura.

A small pneumothorax may not be visualized on routine films, but can usually be identified if the radiograph is taken in expiration (Figure 8.14). Large pneumothoraces are obvious on clinical grounds and there is no difficulty in confirming the diagnosis from the radiograph.

A tension pneumothorax cannot be diagnosed by plain films alone—mediastinal shift and downward displacement of the diaphragm do not necessarily indicate a high intrathoracic pressure. It is important to realise that a tension pneumothorax may be of only moderate size and there may be no diaphragmatic displacement.

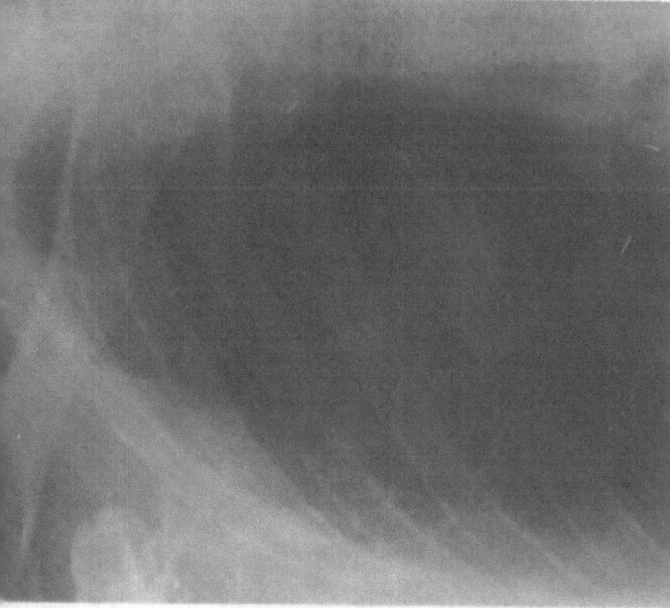

Figure 8.12. *Upper zone mass on PA radiograph. Note the destruction of the anterior end of the adjacent rib. Myeloma.*

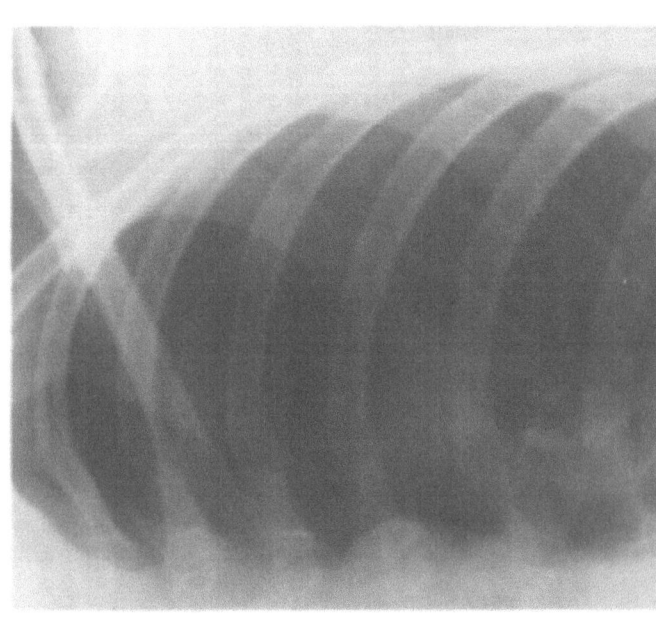

Figure 8.14. *Small pneumothorax which was only visible on this expiratory film.*

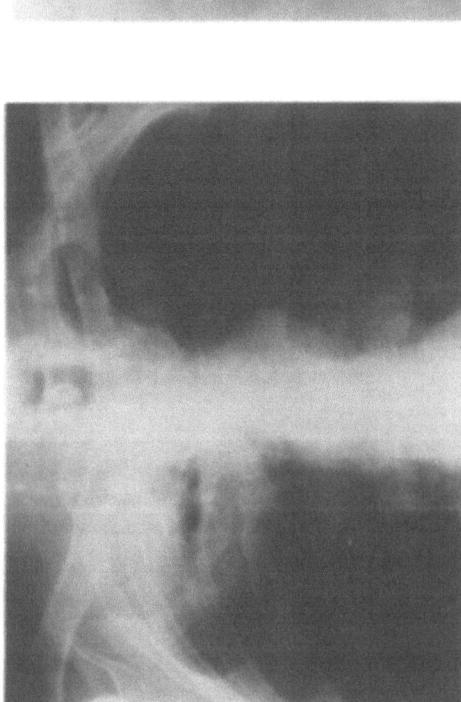

Figure 8.13. *Cavitating mass at the apex of the right lung which has destroyed the adjacent first rib. Pancoast tumour. (Courtesy of Dr J.E. Williams.)*

Small and large pneumothoraces may be simulated by bullae. Fine strands extending across the transradiant area and demarcating the edge of the bullae sometimes allow the differentiation to be made (Figure 8.15). If a pneumothorax is mistakenly diagnosed and the lesion intubated, a persistent air leak may ensue.

Very rarely a pneumothorax may present with subcutaneous emphysema. However, the association of pleural air or fluid and subcutaneous air should suggest the possibility of a bronchial or oesophageal tear. Both are important complications of blunt chest trauma, whilst the latter may occur spontaneously or as a complication of endoscopy.

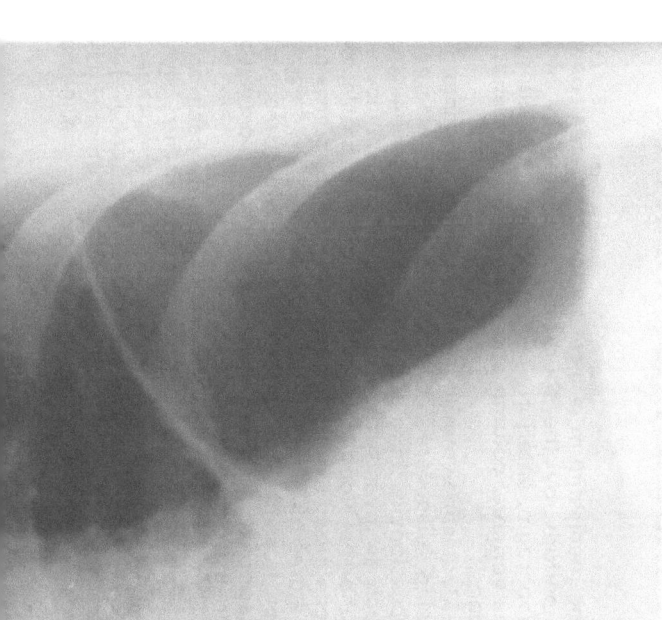

Figure 8.15. Large bullae at the left base. It is often difficult to differentiate these from a pneumothorax. Note the fine septa delineating the wall of the bulla.

9. Mediastinal Masses

The mediastinum is a relatively small area bounded superiorly by the thoracic inlet, inferiorly by the diaphragm, anteriorly by the sternum, posteriorly by the vertebral column and laterally by the pleura and lungs.

Mediastinal masses are frequently asymptomatic, being discovered on routine chest radiographs. Occasionally there are clinical clues to the diagnosis, such as myasthenia gravis with thymic tumours, an abnormal blood count in leukaemia or neuroblastoma, generalized lymphadenopathy with lymphomas or the features of an aortic aneurysm. While it is frequently not possible to establish a definite preoperative diagnosis, radiology probably offers the most valuable means to that end.

Some mediastinal masses are only seen on the lateral film which is the most important film, because it allows one to localize accurately a mass seen on the PA projection. Localization is important in predicting the nature of the mass, as certain tumours have a predilection for particular areas within the mediastinum.

While plain radiography is usually sufficient to demonstrate a lesion, tomography is sometimes required for better definition of the lesion. Fluoroscopy is occasionally valuable, particularly in infants, in differentiating a normal thymus from a pathological mass. It is of limited value in the diagnosis of aneurysms, because tumours adjacent to the aorta and main pulmonary arteries exhibit transmitted pulsation which is difficult to differentiate from the intrinsic pulsation of aneurysms. Oesophageal lesions are diagnosed by means of a barium swallow. Computerized tomography provides an excellent means of imaging the mediastinum. It sorts out the questionably abnormal mediastinum, accurately determines tumour site and extent and allows a specific diagnosis in certain circumstances, e.g. aneurysms.

The mediastinum may be divided into four major components with reference to the lateral film. The anterior mediastinum lies anterior to the heart; the middle mediastinum is largely occupied by the heart and great vessels, together with the major bronchi; the posterior mediastinum extends from the posterior aspect of the heart to the vertebrae and ribs; and the superior mediastinum is that area above an arbitrary line drawn from the upper end of the sternum to the fifth dorsal vertebra.

It is appropriate to consider the lesions according to their anatomical site.

Anterior Mediastinal Masses

Small anterior mediastinal masses are usually invisible on the routine PA projections, therefore a lateral film is mandatory. Coned views with the arms well up or back are useful, and tomography is often very rewarding. The outstanding abnormality is a loss of the normal retrosternal translucency. More superior lesions may displace the trachea. The more common anterior mediastinal masses are listed in Table 9.1.

Table 9.1. Anterior mediastinal masses.

Retrosternal thyroid
Dermoid (teratoma)
Thymic masses (thymoma; cyst)
Lymphomas
Aortic aneurysm
Tumours of the sternum
Pericardial cyst
Morgagni hernia
Ectopic thyroid or parathyroid glands
Tortuous innominate artery

Retrosternal goitres are seen high in the anterior mediastinum, extending into or from the superior mediastinum (Figure 9.1). The trachea is commonly displaced, and at fluoroscopy the opacity moves with swallowing. Calcification is frequently present and does not differentiate a benign from a malignant

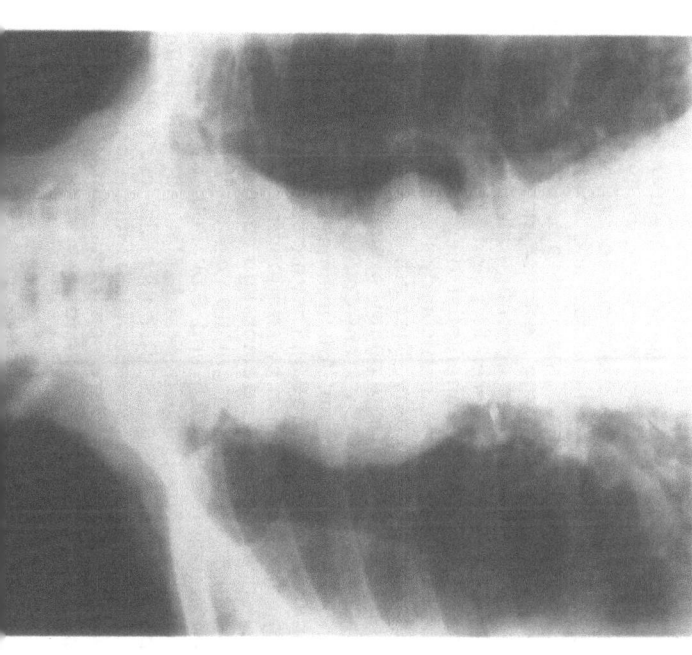

Figure 9.1. *Large retrosternal goitre with characteristic displacement of the trachea.*

goitre. The lesion may be mimicked in elderly patients by a tortuous innominate artery or the much rarer innominate artery aneurysm.

Dermoids and thymic tumours are usually centrally situated in the anterior mediastinum, lying adjacent to the aortic root or main pulmonary artery (Figure 9.2). They are of variable size and both may calcify. Lateral tomography is required to demonstrate small tumours, whilst large lesions may produce an apparently bizarre cardiac configuration on the PA film. Aneurysms of the ascending aorta must always be considered in the differential diagnosis of anterior mediastinal masses, particularly those overlying the right pulmonary artery. They are not always calcified and frequently pulsate poorly, which belies the value of fluoroscopy. If there is any doubt, CT or aortography should be performed. Aneurysms of the pulmonary artery are rare (Figure 9.3). They are distinguished from an adjacent neoplasm by arteriography.

Pericardial cysts and diaphragmatic hernias through the foramen of Morgagni are very similar in appearance (Figures 9.4, 9.5 and 9.6). Both must be distinguished from large pericardial fat pads. Ultrasound permits the diagnosis of pericardial cysts. Hernias frequently contain omentum (a barium enema usually reveals upward displacement of the transverse colon) or liver, which is confirmed by a radionuclide liver scan.

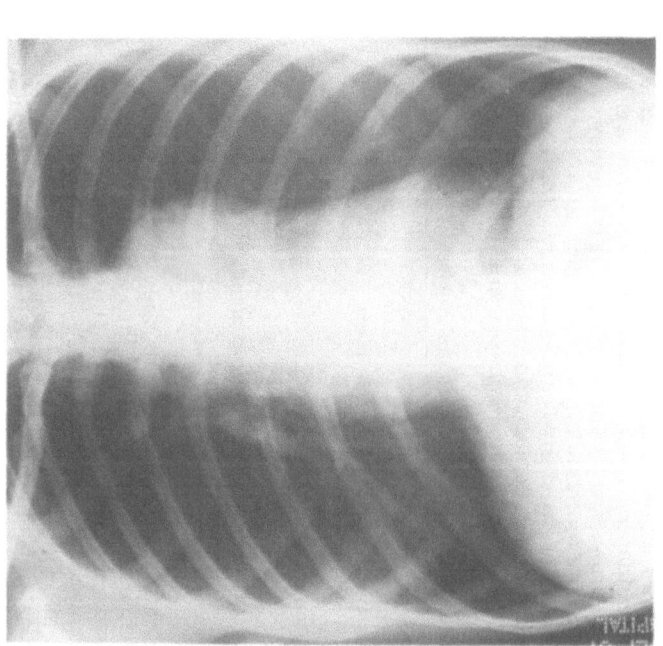

Figure 9.2. *Dermoid overlying the pulmonary artery. A thymic tumour might give rise to an identical appearance.*

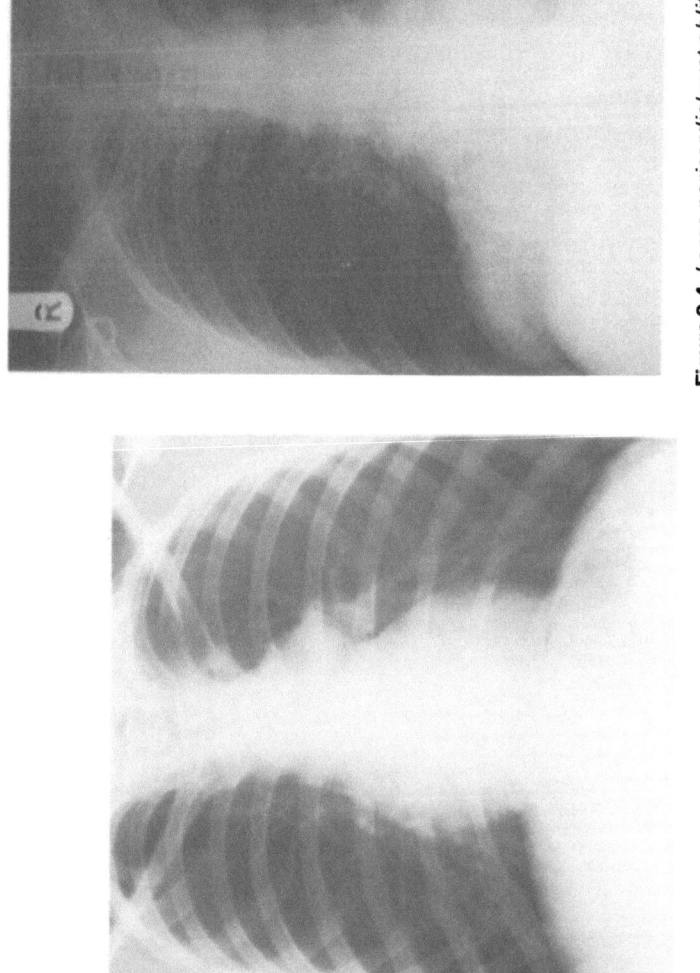

Figure 9.3. Aneurysm of the pulmonary artery.

Figure 9.4. Large pericardial cyst obliterating the right cardio-phrenic angle.

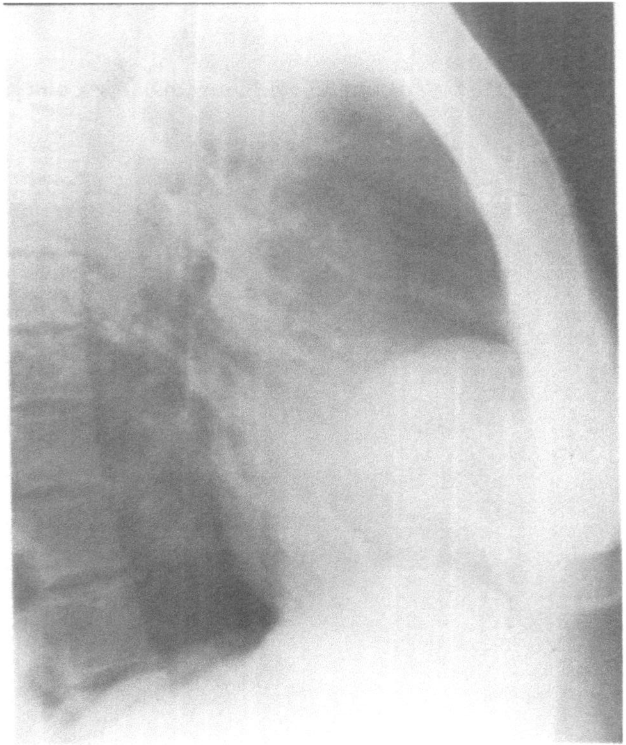

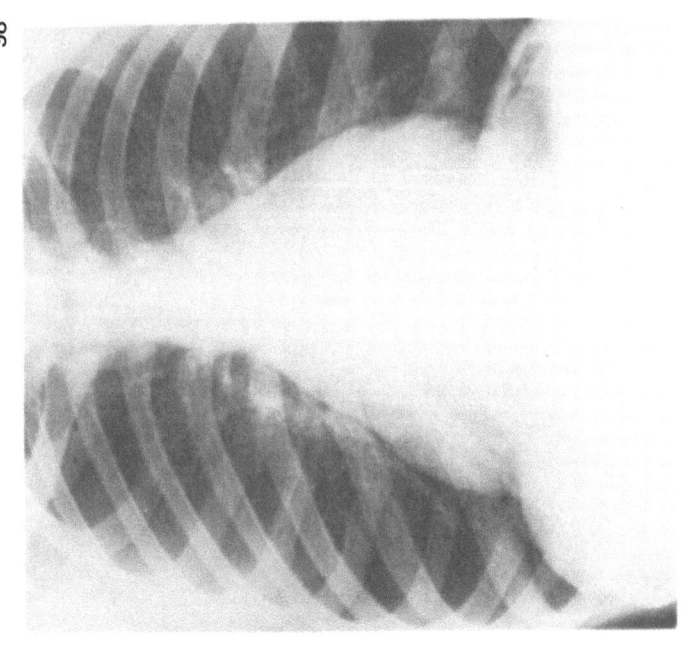

Figure 9.5. Lateral view of Figure 9.4.

Figure 9.6. Morgagni hernia. The appearances are suggestive of a pericardial cyst. The hernia contained liver.

Lymphomas and leukaemia occasionally present with retrosternal deposits which may be quite large. Leukaemia is probably the commonest cause of an anterior mediastinal mass in a child.

Primary or secondary tumours of the sternum are extremely rare. They are distinguished from non-bony masses by attention to the sternum on the lateral film.

Middle Mediastinal Masses

Most middle mediastinal masses are caused by enlarged lymph nodes. These lie in the paratracheal, tracheobronchial, bronchopulmonary (hilar) and subcarinal situations. Such lymphadenopathy may be caused by neoplastic involvement, sarcoidosis or a chronic inflammatory process.

Table 9.2. Middle mediastinal masses.

Bronchial carcinoma
Lymphomas (Hodgkin's)
Sarcoidosis
Primary tuberculosis
Fungal diseases
Bronchogenic cyst

Table 9.2 lists the commonest lesions, of which a bronchial carcinoma is the most frequent in patients older than 40 years. Hilar enlargement may be assoc-iated with paratracheal and subcarinal node enlargement. The latter occasionally predominates.

Sarcoidosis competes with Hodgkin's disease as the commonest cause of mediastinal lymph node enlargement in younger patients. Bilateral hilar node enlargement occurs in approximately 80 per cent of patients with sarcoidosis with or without pulmonary disease. The lymphadenopathy is nearly always symmetrical (Figure 9.7). Tracheobronchial and paratracheal nodes may be enlarged but rarely in isolation. Again the enlargement is symmetrical. Occasionally right paratracheal adenopathy occurs in isolation, making the differentiation from Hodgkin's disease difficult on radiographic appearances alone. Enlargement of the mediastinal nodes is the most common initial radiographic finding in Hodgkin's disease, occurring in approximately 50 per cent of patients. In contrast to sarcoidosis, the nodal enlargement is frequently asymmetrical. The hilar nodes are spared in about half the patients with mediastinal involvement, and the paratracheal component is often striking (Figure 9.8). Calcification of mediastinal nodes occasionally occurs in both sarcoidosis and Hodgkin's disease, but in the latter only following radiotherapy.

Primary tuberculosis is the commonest inflammatory cause of mediastinal lymphadenopathy. Histoplasmosis and coccidioidomycosis are common in parts of North America. In primary tuberculosis there is

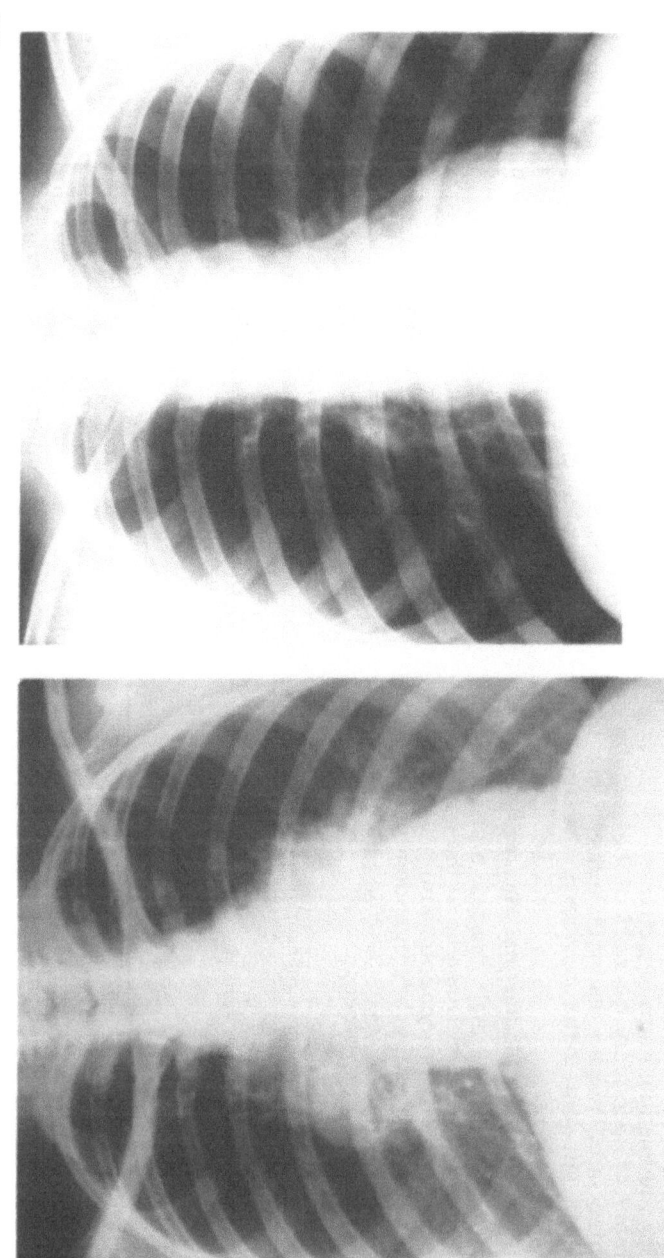

Figure 9.7. Sarcoidosis. Bilateral symmetrical hilar lymphadenopathy.

Figure 9.8. Hodgkin's disease. Marked paratracheal node enlargement with sparing of the hila.

often some associated pulmonary shadowing; this diagnosis should be especially remembered in patients who are recent immigrants to the UK (Figure 9.9).

Bronchogenic cysts lie adjacent to the major bronchi. They may be subcarinal in position and on tomography they are well defined. They are usually asymptomatic.

Posterior Mediastinal Masses

The commoner posterior mediastinal lesions are listed in Table 9.3.

Table 9.3. Posterior mediastinal masses.

Neurogenic tumours
    Neurilemmoma
    Ganglioneuroma
    Neuroblastoma
    Phaeochromocytoma
Meningocoele
Paravertebral abscess
Paravertebral tumour extension
Paravertebral haematoma
Oesophageal lesions
Aortic aneurysm

Neurogenic tumours are the most frequent lesions in this group. They lie in the costovertebral gutter and arise from the sympathetic chain and from the inter-costal nerves (Figures 9.10 and 9.11) and may cause

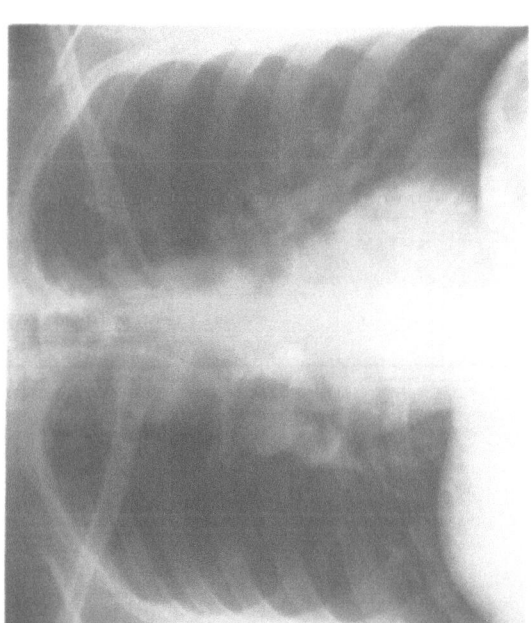

Figure 9.9. *Tuberculosis. Right hilar and paratracheal lympha-denopathy.*

erosion of the adjacent vertebral body or ribs. Both benign and malignant lesions may calcify. Careful inspection of the vertebral bodies is important in deciding whether there is any intraspinal extension of

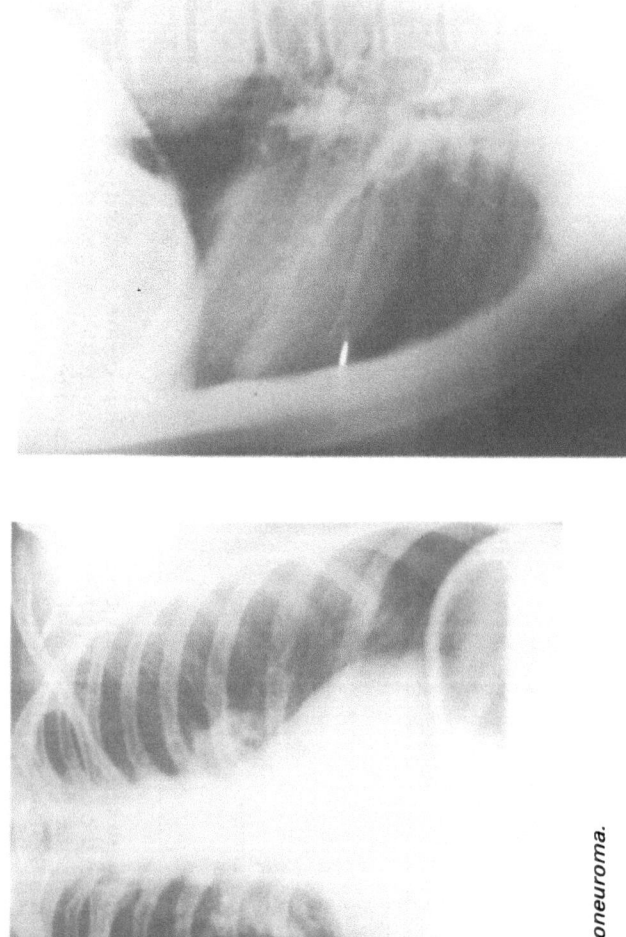

Figure 9.10. *Ganglioneuroma.*

Figure 9.11. *Lateral film of the same patient as Figure 9.10 confirms the posterior position of the mass.*

the lesion or, conversely, whether the lesion has arisen from the spinal column. Tomography can be very helpful and myelography may be required. Thoracic meningocoeles are rare. They occur in association with spinal dysraphism and usually as part of the general complex of neurofibromatosis.

A dilated oesophagus, such as occurs in achalasia, may present as a mediastinal mass (Figure 9.12). It usually extends to the right on the PA film, and the retrocardiac area is obliterated by a characteristic mottled opacity caused by a combination of food and air. Pulmonary changes from recurrent overspill pneumonitis may be evident.

Neoplasms arising from the oesophagus and gastroenteric cysts are rare abnormalities. Their diagnosis is usually apparent on a barium swallow. Diaphragmatic hernias are very common causes of a retrocardiac opacity; the appearance is typical and the diagnosis is usually obvious from the lateral film.

A paravertebral mass is associated with spinal malignancy (especially metastases) with an inflammatory spondylitis and with vertebral fractures. Such a mass may first be seen in the lower dorsal region on a well-penetrated PA film taken for referred chest pain (Figure 9.13). Coned views and tomograms are required to distinguish these conditions. The intervertebral disc spaces are usually narrowed and eroded by an inflammatory process, in contrast to the destruction of the vertebral body or pedicles by metastases.

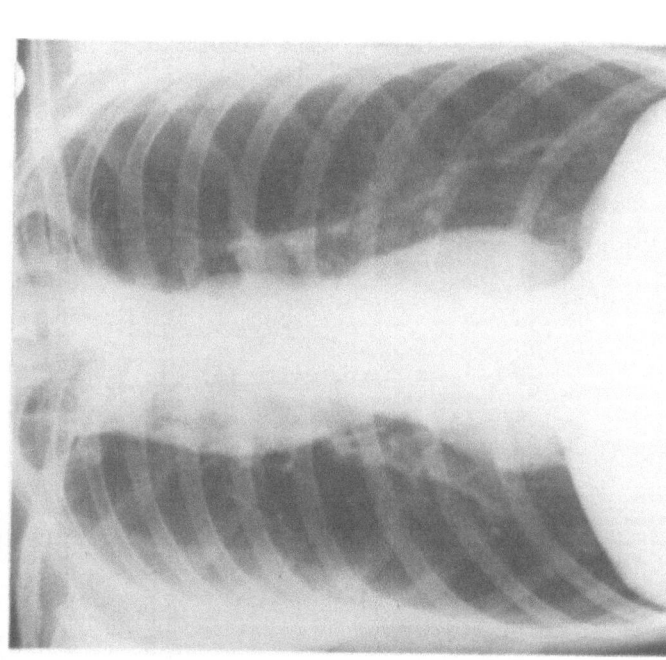

Figure 9.12. Achalasia. The dilated oesophagus widens the mediastinum. Note the absence of air in the gastric fundus.

103

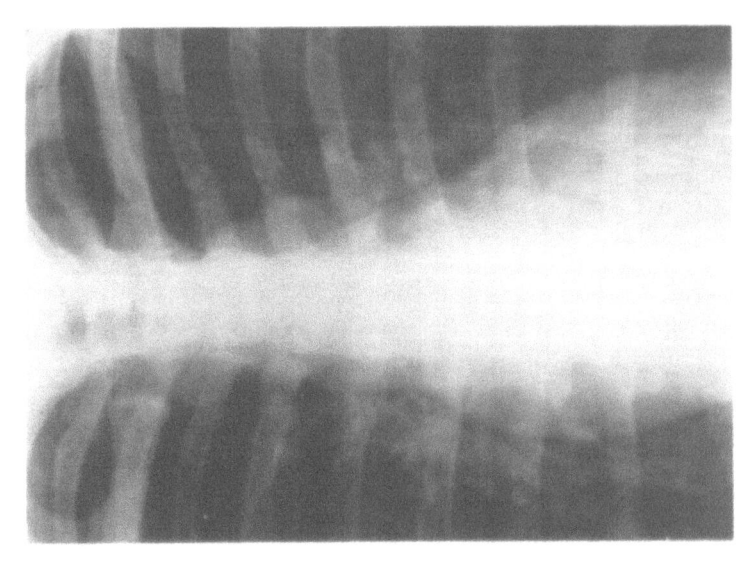

Figure 9.13. *Tuberculous spondylitis producing a paravertebral soft tissue mass.*

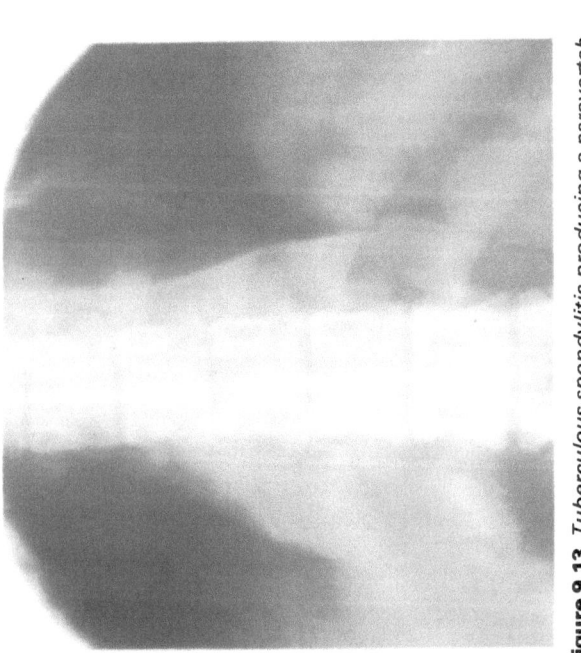

Figure 9.14. *Abnormal shadow at the aortic knuckle. (Courtesy of Dr G. Verney.)*

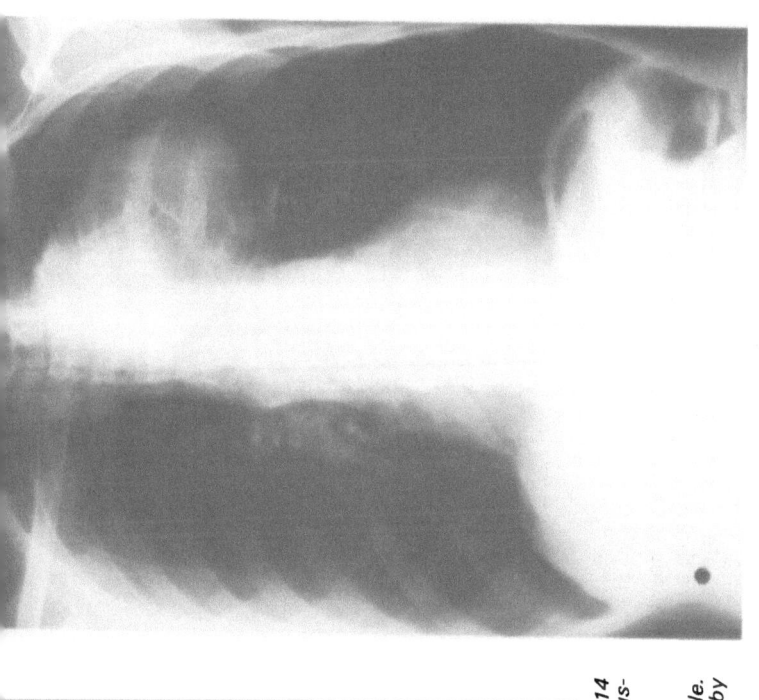

Figure 9.15. Aortogram of the same patient as in Figure 9.14 reveals an aneurysm at the aortic arch. The patient had sustained blunt trauma to the chest six months previously.

Figure 9.16. Large mass obliterating the aortic knuckle. Bronchial carcinoma. Aneurysm suspected but excluded by aortography.

As in the anterior mediastinum, aortic aneurysms (whether simple or of the dissecting variety) are great mimics of all the previously mentioned tumours. They may especially simulate the neurogenic tumours, causing similar rib and vertebral body erosion. It is advisable to perform CT and/or aortography in cases where there is any doubt as to the nature of the lesion (Figures 9.14 to 9.16).

10. The Diaphragm

The diaphragm is a musculotendinous sheet which separates the thoracic from the abdominal contents. Variations in its position, movement or appearance are fairly common and may serve to establish the presence and occasionally the nature of abnormalities in both the chest and the abdomen.

In most people the right leaf of the diaphragm lies at a slightly higher level than the left leaf. This is related to the presence of the heart rather than the liver, as in dextroversion without situs inversus the left leaf lies at a higher level than the right leaf. Both leaves normally move fairly equally over 2 to 3 cm during forced respiration. With sniffing, an even greater amplitude of movement may be seen. However, in approximately five per cent of normal patients, paradoxical (upward) movement may occur with this manoeuvre, which accordingly cannot be used as a diagnostic test of phrenic paralysis.

It is important to be conversant with some normal variations in diaphragmatic contour. A common appearance is a hump-shaped deformity at the

anteromedial aspect of the right hemidiaphragm (Figure 10.1). This may simulate, for example, an anterior mediastinal hernia or a pericardial cyst. It is probably due to a local congenital deficiency of musculature at this site and is frequently termed a cupola or local eventration. Less commonly the muscular deficiency extends over a greater area, involving most of the anterior aspect of the right hemidiaphragm. On a single PA film this resembles an elevated diaphragm (Figures 10.2 and 10.3).

Eventration is a congenital abnormality in which there is complete absence of musculature. It almost always affects the left leaf, which appears high and exhibits paradoxical movement at fluoroscopy. It is impossible to differentiate eventration from phrenic nerve palsy unless serial films are available. It almost certainly accounts for some causes of idiopathic left diaphragmatic paralysis.

Gaseous distension of the stomach occasionally causes slight elevation or an unusual configuration of the left leaf. Colonic interposition may occur on the right (Figure 10.4).

Diaphragmatic Hernias

By far the commonest diaphragmatic hernia occurs at the oesophagogastric hiatus. Large hiatal hernias occur, particularly in the elderly (see Figure 1.3) where

107

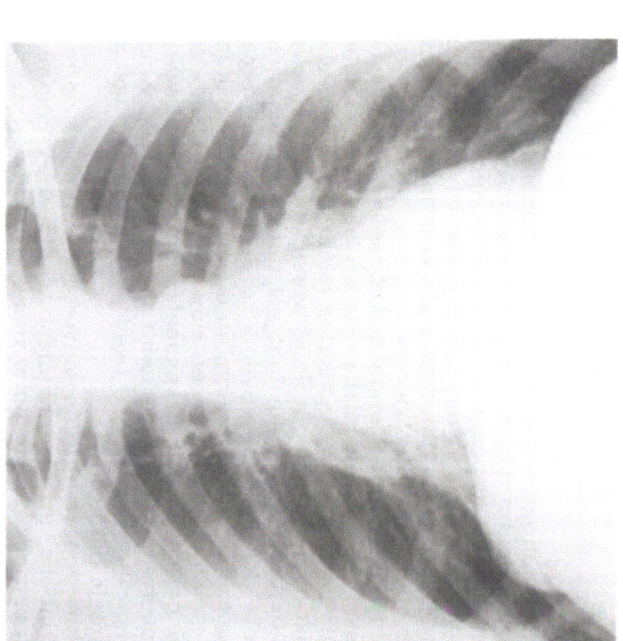

Figure 10.1. Characteristic hump-shaped deformity at the anteromedial aspect of the right hemidiaphragm due to a local muscular deficiency.

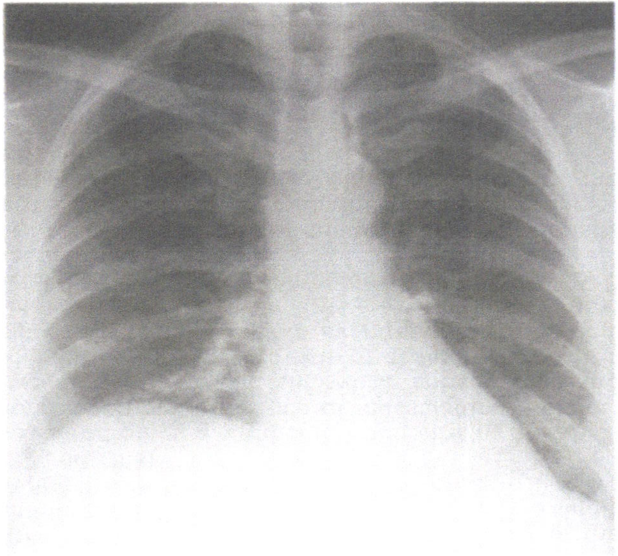

Figure 10.2. The right leaf of the diaphragm appears elevated on the PA projection.

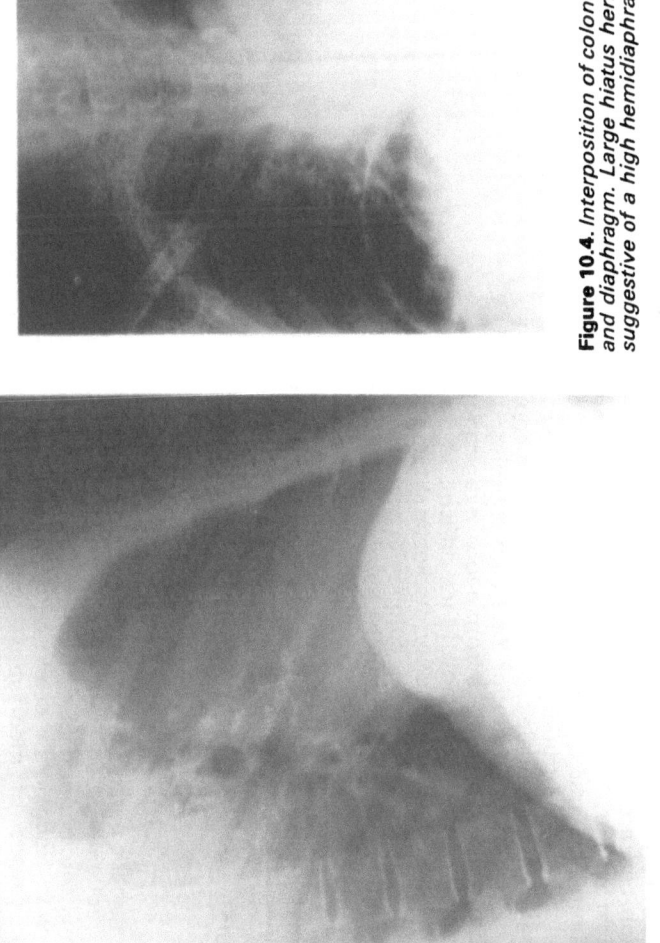

Figure 10.3. The lateral film confirms that this is simply due to a muscular deficiency of its anterior portion. Note that both costovertebral angles lie at the same level.

Figure 10.4. Interposition of colon on the right, between liver and diaphragm. Large hiatus hernia of the left superficially suggestive of a high hemidiaphragm.

109

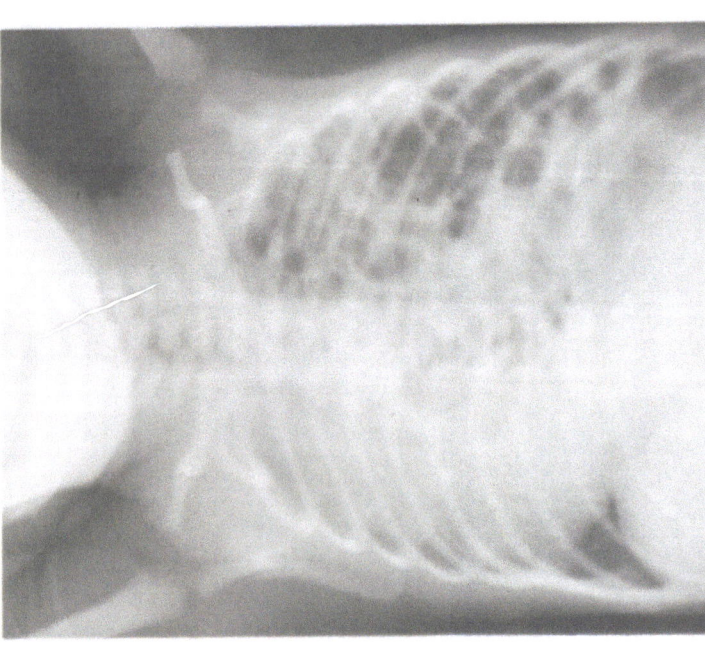

Figure 10.5. *Congenital diaphragmatic hernia. Air-filled gut fills the left hemithorax.*

a large retrocardiac shadow, frequently containing a fluid level, may be seen on PA and lateral projections. Diaphragmatic hernias in the neonatal period are a common cause of respiratory distress (Figure 10.5). The chest may be filled with gut, allowing the abdomen to assume its characteristic scaphoid appearance.

Local hernias protruding through the foramina of Morgagni and Bochdalek are occasionally encountered in adulthood. Anterior Morgagni hernias are often difficult to differentiate from a local eventration, although this is unimportant. More difficult is their differentiation from low anterior mediastinal tumours (see Figure 9.6). Either liver or colon with accompanying omentum, extends through the hernia. A liver scan or barium enema establishes the diagnosis.

Bochdalek hernias often contain only fat, but occasionally contain organs such as the kidney. It is important to establish the extrapulmonary nature of the opacity which may otherwise be mistaken for an intrapulmonary mass.

Diaphragmatic Paralysis

Diaphragmatic paralysis due to phrenic nerve palsy is most frequently seen with mediastinal spread of bronchial carcinoma (Figure 10.6). It is seldom associated with Hodgkin's disease or with other, more benign, causes of mediastinal lymphadenopathy, such as sarcoidosis. Phrenic palsy is sometimes observed following cervical sympathectomy, while in the past it was the natural accompaniment of phrenic crush for tuberculosis. It is occasionally seen with such rarities as a mediastinal abscess or leaking aortic aneurysm. Unexplained instances of phrenic nerve palsy are common and are possibly related to a viral neuritis. They almost invariably occur on the right.

Subphrenic Abscesses

A subphrenic abscess often causes elevation of the adjacent hemidiaphragm. A pleural effusion of variable size is a frequent accompaniment, and inhibition of diaphragmatic movement is common. However, diaphragmatic elevation with partial paralysis may occur with pleurisy, lower lobe pneumonia, or following an episode of pulmonary infarction. It is therefore necessary, when attempting to establish the diagnosis of a subphrenic abscess, to identify any gas or fluid level within the abscess (Figure 10.7). Well penetrated coned views of the upper abdomen, in erect, supine and lateral projections, are useful in this respect (Figures 10.8 and 10.9).

All too frequently the diagnosis cannot be established by radiographic means. It is in these instances that ultrasound and computerized tomography are most useful.

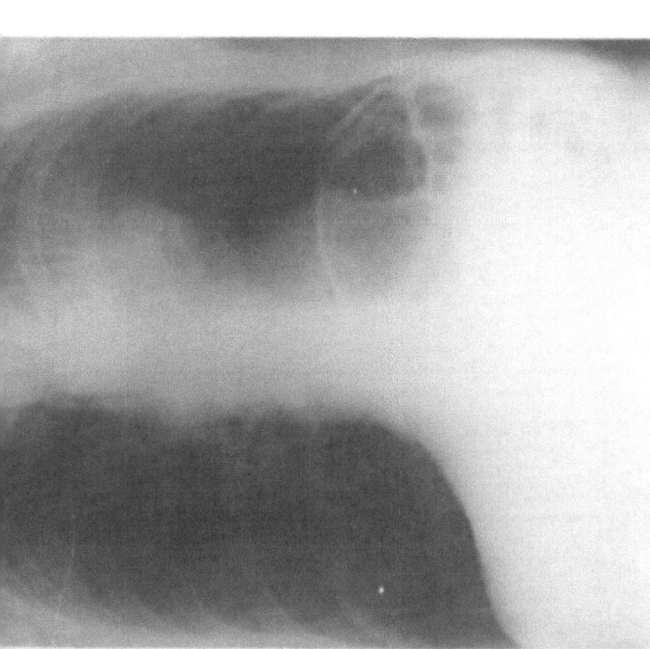

Figure 10.6. Bronchial carcinoma causing left upper lobe collapse and phrenic nerve palsy, with resultant elevation of the left hemidiaphragm.

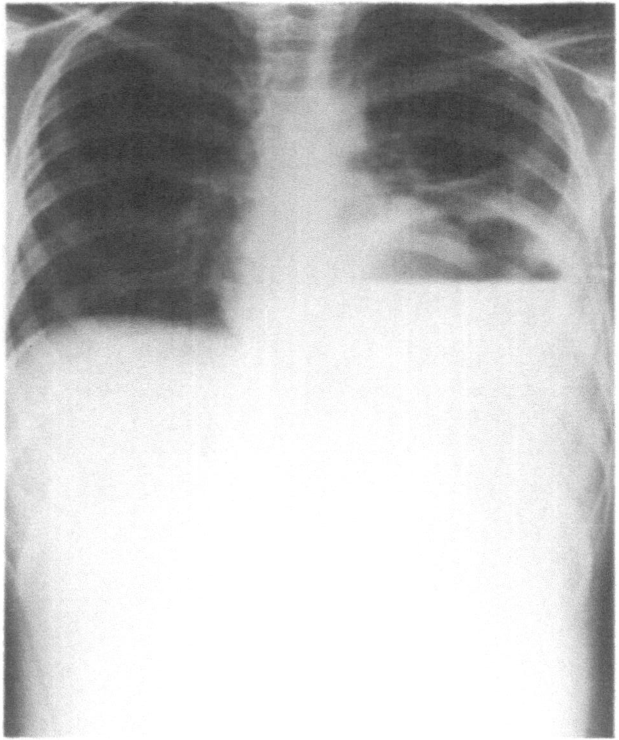

Figure 10.7. A large left subphrenic abscess superficially resembling gastric distension.

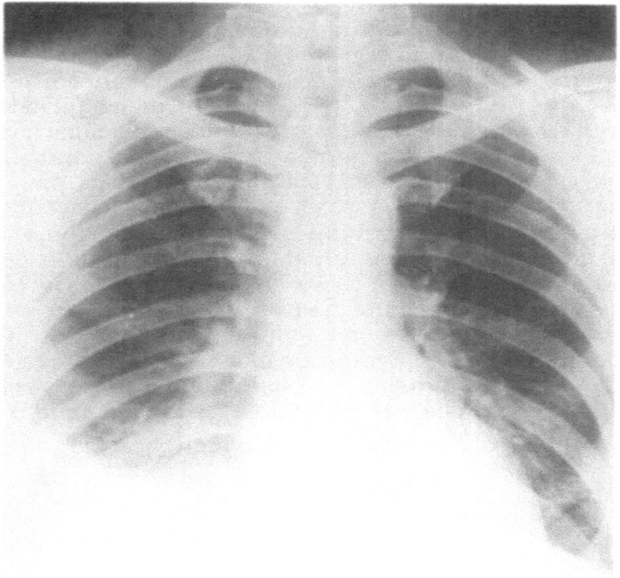

Figure 10.8. An under-exposed film in a patient suspected of having a subphrenic abscess reveals a right pleural effusion.

Elevation of the diaphragm may be simulated by a sharply marginated opacity in the adjacent pleura or lung. Subpulmonary collections of pleural fluid, in particular, may produce an appearance similar to diaphragmatic elevation. Films taken with the patient in the supine or decubitus position will allow the pleural fluid to extend in a cephalad direction. The diaphragm can then be identified and will be seen to lie in its normal position (Figures 10.10 and 10.11). Less commonly a large mass in the lower lobe, or combined right middle and lower lobe collapse, will suggest a peculiar diaphragmatic contour with elevation (Figure 10.12).

Rupture of the Diaphragm

Rupture of the diaphragm is more common on the left than on the right side (Figure 10.13). Herniation of the stomach or bowel may occur, even through a small vent, and torsion of the gut, with the formation of an obstructed closed loop, is a serious complication. This serves to emphasize the importance of distinguishing this condition from an eventration or diaphragmatic paralysis. The diagnosis should be suspected following blunt chest trauma when there is an unusual diaphragmatic configuration or an unexplained pleural effusion or fluid level (Figure 10.14).

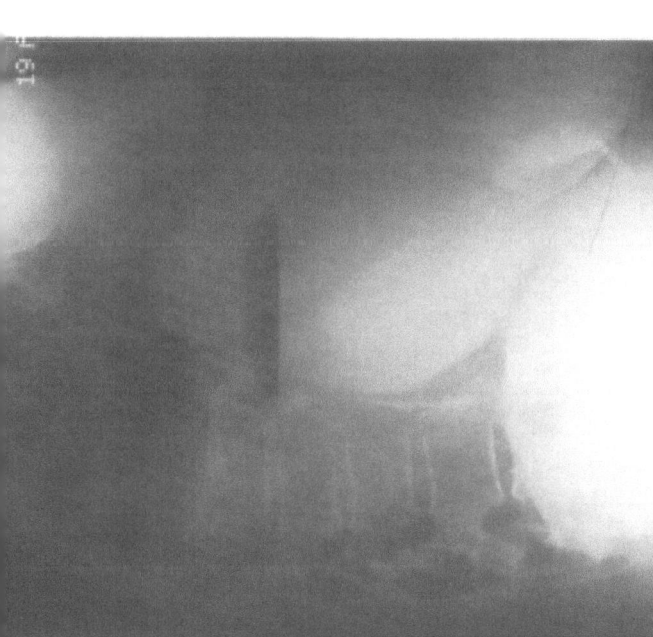

Figure 10.9. An erect, well penetrated lateral film reveals a fluid level within a large subphrenic abscess cavity.

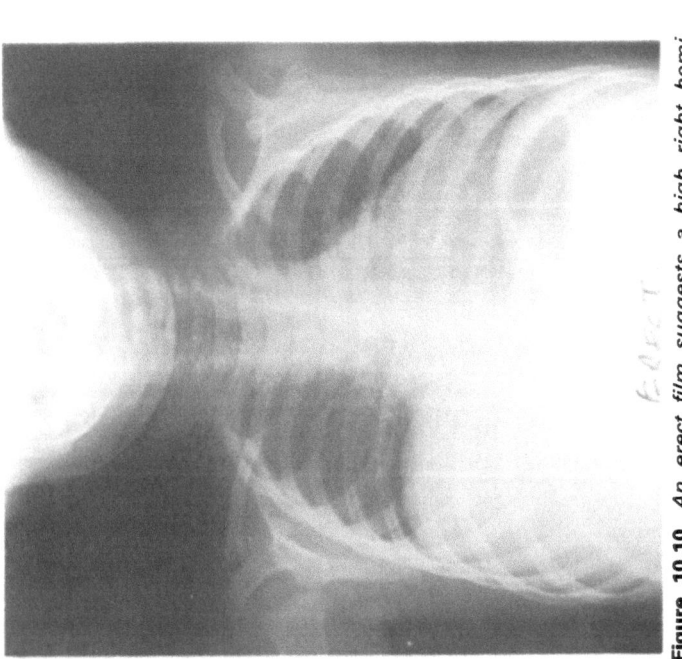

Figure 10.10. An erect film suggests a high right hemidiaphragm.

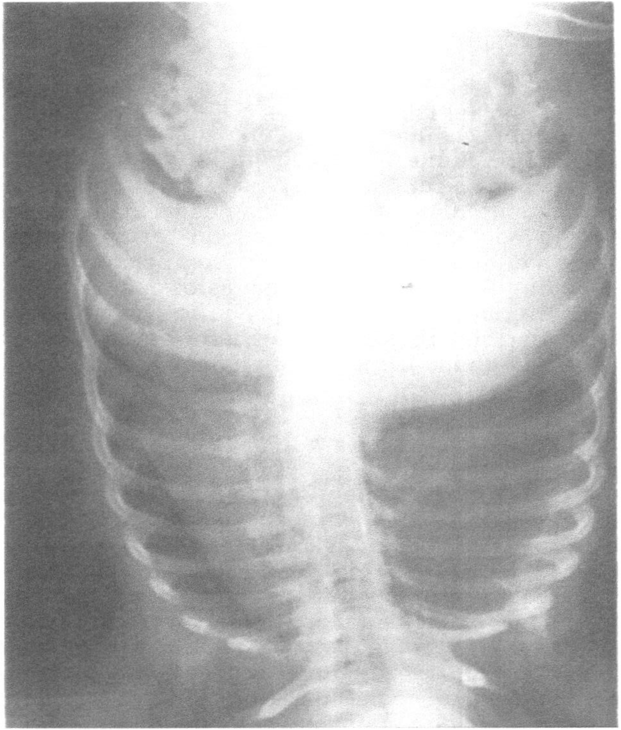

Figure 10.11. A film taken with the patient supine establishes the normal position of the diaphragm. The pleural fluid now lies posteriorly behind the right lung.

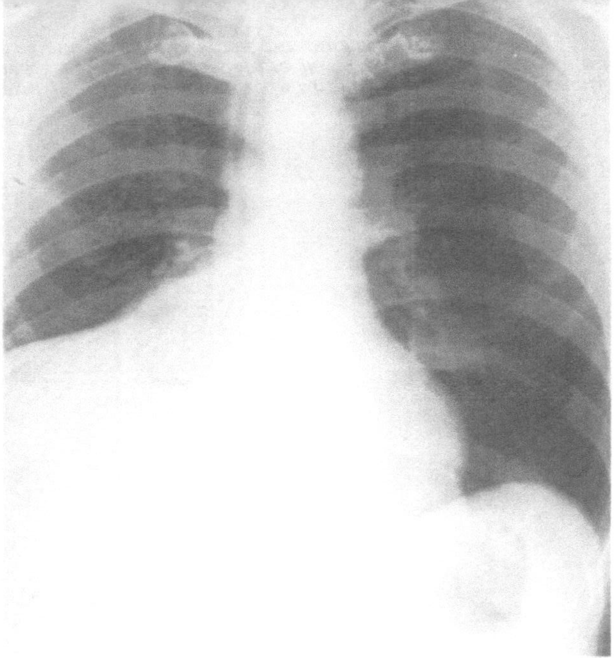

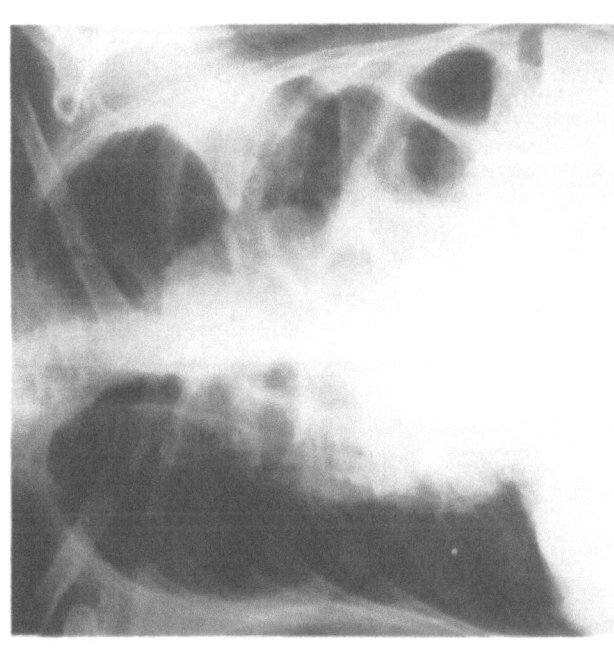

Figure 10.12. Right middle and lower lobe collapse. The appearances superficially resemble an abnormally positioned diaphragm.

Figure 10.13. Herniation of small bowel through a long standing and previously undiagnosed tear in the left leaf of the diaphragm. The patient presented with acute intestinal obstruction.

115

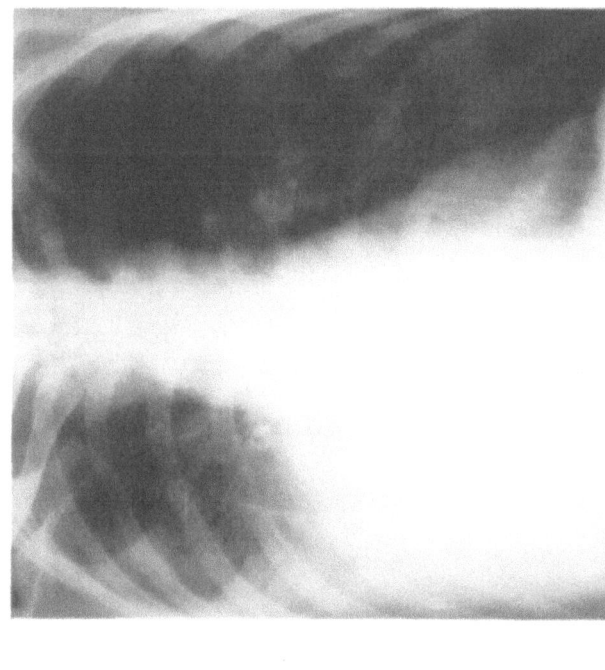

Figure 10.15. Rupture of the right leaf of the diaphragm following a road traffic accident. The findings are non-specific. The diagnosis requires a high index of suspicion. A diagnostic pneumoperitoneum may be useful.

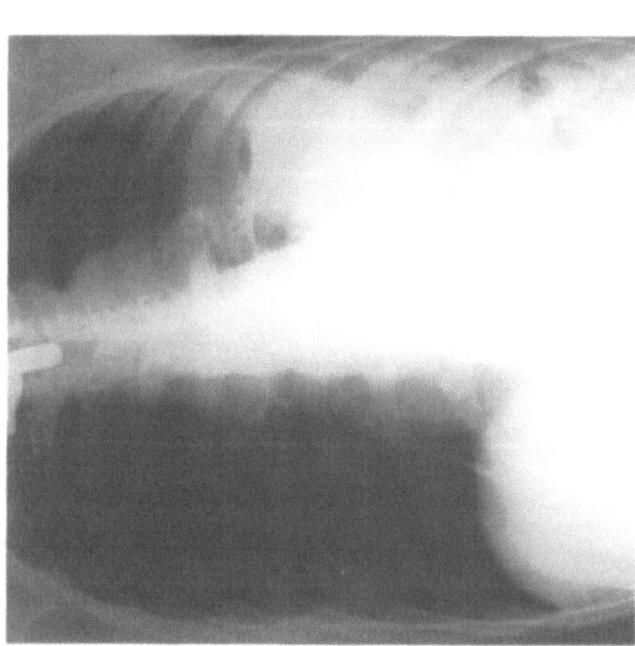

Figure 10.14. Rupture of the left hemidiaphragm. An opacity obliterates the left leaf. There is an effusion and herniated gut as shown by the small gas pocket and fluid level.

The diagnosis can usually be established quite readily on the left by means of a contrast study with barium given either by mouth or as an enema. It is much more difficult to prove the diagnosis of a rup-tured right hemidiaphragm (Figure 10.15). If a pneumo-peritoneum is induced, the air will usually extend via the tear to the pleural space with a resultant pneumo-thorax.

Index